A Note on Confidentiality

This book is rooted in real events and personal experiences. However, patient and staff confidentiality is paramount.

To protect the integrity of clinical practice and the privacy of those involved, all names, identifying characteristics, and specific details (including hospitals, trusts, and geographical locations) have been changed, obscured, or fictionalised.

Furthermore, this narrative is a synthesis. While it follows my personal journey, it incorporates the documented realities and shared debriefs of the student nurses and clinicians who occupied these spaces with me. In certain cases, a degree of creative license has been employed: chronologies have been compressed, dialogue has been reconstructed, and amalgam characters have been created to better illustrate the recurring patterns of the modern healthcare environment.

I had many mentors, more than one boyfriend (albeit one at a time), and the occasional predator who mistook my silence for permission: identify yourself at your peril. You are seeing a mosaic of a systemic reality any attempt to map these composite characters onto specific individuals is structurally impossible. Any resemblance to actual persons living or dead, is purely coincidental.

The priority of **Unvarnished Press** is to preserve the clinical, emotional, and institutional truth of these experiences. This is an archive of the front line, documented to ensure that the realities of the profession are brought into the light.

This book is for educational and entertainment purposes only and does not constitute medical advice or professional nursing instruction.

Signed:

An unashamedly, currently suspended Nurse.

ROOKIE NURSES: BUCKLE UP

VICTORIA HINDS

ROOKIE NURSES: BUCKLE UP
Student Edition

The grit, wit and weight of the ward

An |UP| Ltd Publication

|UP|
UNVARNISHED PRESS
—

First published in Great Britain in 2026 by Unvarnished Press

A CIP catalogue record for this book is available from the British Library.

ISBN: 978-1-9195144-0-6

Typeset by Unvarnished Press
Printed and bound in Great Britain by Amazon/KDP

For The Boy
the very reason I exist.

For My Person
who has lived every second of triumph and trauma with me.

For The Rentals
for getting me through. Sorry I couldn't stay quiet.

Contents

Foreword

If you bought this book looking for a heartwarming tale about the "calling" of nursing, do us both a favour and put it back on the shelf. There are plenty of memoirs out there that focus on the grace of the profession, and I don't begrudge them their perspective; we all needed a way to cope with the madness. But this isn't one of those stories. You won't find any "angels" here. Angels have wings; back then, I had a landlord who didn't answer the phone, a teenage son who spent the equivalent of an annual holiday on scooter parts, and a recurring nightmare about being struck off in my first week because I was nothing but an imposter in a uniform.

I didn't enter the nursing profession because I had a surplus of energy or a martyr complex. I entered it because life had already shown me its sharp edges, and I figured if I was going to stand in the fire, I might as well learn how to put it out. My resilience wasn't a personality trait. It was a survival mechanism, forged in the heat of panic and the cold reality of a student bursary that disappeared faster than a box of chocolates in a staff room.

Back then, I was living on the breadline, studying full-time and working full-time, somehow inhabiting a world where there were suddenly twenty-eight hours in a day, every single day. I couldn't even complain about the cost of those scooter parts; those two wheels were the only reason The Boy made it to school on time while I was busy trying to find the mental bandwidth to function on four hours of sleep and a diet of sheer tenacity.

The 21st-century student nurse is a strange creature. We are the ghosts of the ward, expected to possess the clinical knowledge of a registrar and the stamina of a pack mule, all while being told our "learning" was the priority as we emptied a commode that had seen better decades. We live in the gap between the policy and the reality. The policy says we should have an hour for lunch; the reality is a cereal bar eaten over a clinical waste bin while contemplating the life choices that led us to this specific corridor.

There was a certain kind of humour that grew in the dark corners of those hospitals. It was the kind of laugh that sounded a bit like a sob if you listen too closely. It was the jokes we told to keep the darkness at bay when a shift felt like an uphill sprint in lead boots. If you find the contents of these pages raw, it's because the reality of the front line didn't leave much room for varnish. For us, the absurdity was the only thing that kept the trauma from sinking its teeth in.

I remember my first day on placement. I arrived with a pen that worked and a soul that hadn't yet been marinated in the scent of pseudomonas and the heavy, grey fog of a double shift. By midday, I had lost the pen, and by the end of the week, I realised that the system was held together not by the taxpayer's hard-earned contribution or "heroism," but by a thin, straining line of burnt-out humans who were simply too tired to quit; mostly because the promised corporate handshake at the end of it all was just golden enough to keep us tethered to the madness.

This book is the record of that struggle. It is for the mothers who study anatomy at the kitchen table while their children sleep. It is for the students who cry in the car before a shift because the thought of another twelve hours of "unpaid learning" feels like a prison sentence. It is for anyone who has ever felt the silence of a hospital corridor at 4:00 AM and wondered if they had anything left to give.

Don't expect a hero's journey. There was no grand epiphany at the end of the corridor. There was only the next shift, the next patient, and the heavy, rhythmic thud of the security door locking behind me.

Buckle up.

How to Be a Student Nurse and

Survive What You Do Not Talk About

I promised myself that day would be the first day. The first day I actually turned up. I wanted to be present, engaged, and perhaps even eager to begin the gruelling evolution toward becoming Nurse Hinds. However, personal circumstances, specifically the volatile breakdown of the relationship I was in days before day one, meant that just functioning was an effort that took great mental preparation.

This was the man I had introduced to The Boy. I had allowed him into our personal space and honestly thought I would spend the rest of my life with him. He was also the man who knocked my tooth out, split my lip open, and attempted to strangle me after a night out on the booze. I later found out that he moved in with me not because of his declared undying love, but because he had been evicted from his last rental. A caravan.

It transpired that he did not enjoy anything about living with me. He was in a permanent state of anger as he missed the daily carvery, the regular karaoke, and purchasing a pint for less than in a Wetherspoons at the shithole; I rephrase, the campsite he used to reside on.

I had believed he lived in a beautiful five-bedroom cottage that I visited often. It turned out he had it all timed very well, and the house belonged to a relative. We only stayed there when that relative was at work away. My red flag radar was far from operable; it was buried in a shallow grave next to my self-respect. Sympathetic overdrive and necessity were the only things getting me out the door.

I managed to get my sorry arse up and out of bed looking as lively as possible. I was a little less excitable than usual and far from my baseline, but my eyes were open and the lights were on. Unlike most freshers who were still wet behind the ears and going to bed at the same time I was waking up, I had no problem with the early start.

Six years as an agency care assistant had kept me on my toes. The rules of the ward were simple. You report for handover at 07.30 to hit the floor at 08:00. You do not be even a nanosecond late. If you try the "sorry I'm late, I live ages away and traffic was manic" or "I'm a lone parent and my childminder slept in" or even "my car broke down and I've been towed here" excuses, you will get short shrift.

"Report for duty or don't" was the standard response I had been given by most Senior Nurses, irrespective of all personal circumstances. Unless, of course, you are late because your Mum has died or something equally as awful. In those cases, you will be faced with "why the fuck are you here then?" Navigating the nursing mindset is like running a gauntlet. It is a world where empathy is reserved for the patients and the staff are expected to be made of reinforced concrete.

You then finish your shift at 19:30, complete the unpaid handover and exit the building at 20:00. That is only if you are lucky. The bonus of a twelve-hour shift is that you get one fifteen minute and one half hour break. These are strategically placed at intervals when you have no biological need to eat, drink, or piss.

By the time you are finished, you get to do the long drive home and stand semi-comatose under a shower. It might even be a hot one if you can afford the bills. You eat a microwave meal and then pass out dreaming, or nightmaring, of doing it all over.

After the last six years of working in the care sector to test the waters, I had repeatedly hit the glass ceiling. I could go no further in terms of promotion without the credentials. So, it was time for university, round two.

I told myself that if I could survive the brutality of life as an HCA, I could handle Uni. I had done it before; I could do it again. The only difference this time around was that I was almost two decades older and arrived with significantly less enthusiasm. I was there for the qualification and the survival of my household, not the student lifestyle.

Should nursing be an academic degree? That is a topic very much open for debate and one I have many opinions on, but we can chew the fat over that later.

I simply needed that magic piece of paper. I wanted the one with the shiny, embossed seal that deemed you qualified enough to dress a wound and dispense the meds. A few years of hard academic graft seemed a little overzealous for what is essentially a vocational calling, but I was pleased to be able to eventually put letters after my name (maybe).

On day one of my journey, I was already petrified that the process was going to knock the stuffing out of me. I wanted to come out at the end with the same level of passion I went in with. This book, my friends, will tell you if I managed it.

So many people, especially you youngsters, think that university life is there to provide you with good times, drunken laughs, and at least a 2:1 at the end. Many of you live that dream and go on to lead respectable lives. You end up with a mortgage, a couple of kids, an adequate newish car, and a package holiday once a year.

These are all great achievements in the eyes of society. However, you are often the same people who always dreamed of travelling the world, helping others along the way, and making a lasting imprint on humanity itself. You trade the global impact for the safety of a cul-de-sac and a pension. For me, this wasn't about a social calendar or a fresh start in a lecture theatre. It was about securing a future that didn't involve checking the meter every time I wanted to boil the kettle.

I had attempted to gain a degree in the normal order of school, college, and then forcibly committing to a further three years of study. At the time, I chose a subject I had little interest in and possessed a substantial lack of emotional intelligence to realise a vital truth. What you study the first time around is probably the worst decision of your entire life. That decision does not only cuff you with a golden handshake and promises of a fruitful retirement; it cultivates your entire identity.

After not failing, but definitely not achieving my high-functioning capabilities through sheer boredom, I came out of college with a set of A-levels. They were not quite good enough to get into law or politics, so I went through late admissions and chose the degree recommended for my skill set at the time. Who has a skill set at eighteen? I blindly chose from slim pickings based primarily on whether I wanted to live up north or down south.

Real Estate Development and Planning at a riverside campus was the winner. It had a hint of regality about it, so I envisaged a life of pinstripe suits, kitten heels, and reams of contractual fine print. I imagined this would all be broken up with boozy lunches in the city centre and far too many coke-fuelled after-hours parties. It was not until I had to start completing architectural drawings, planning drainage systems, and wearing a hard hat that it dawned on me that probably wasn't the ideal pathway for me.

I decided to flip academia the bird and go it alone. What I had not factored before becoming desperate for a reasonably paid job was that I had entrepreneurial spirit in my blood. I fell into business. I made money; plenty of it. However, I also found a penchant for spending it unscrupulously. I eventually found myself living in a bubble of greed and unfulfillment.

I needed something more. I wanted something meaningful and with a sense of purpose. I craved a life that was less volatile and more stable. Less party hard and more sober on a weekend. So, I walked away from it all. I thought I would try the whole vocational thing to see if I could sleep easier after a day of helping others in their time of need.

I was tired of gauging my level of success based on how much money I had earned, or rather hoodwinked, out of people who, well, really didn't have much money. The transition from a profit margin to a patient's well-being seemed like the only way to burst the bubble I had built for myself.

Coming from a family of nurses, with a father whose career spanned over three decades, I was one of three daughters. I was always told that if any of us were going to follow in his footsteps, it would be me. I was never entirely sure if that was because I displayed innate compassion growing up, or because both of my sisters excelled academically and my parents simply did not think I had it in me.

Either way, I finally stopped ignoring my parents' pleas. After realising that becoming a doctor as a lone parent in my early thirties was most likely way out of reach, nursing it was. To top this process off, university informed me that my A-levels were considered outdated and, worse, in the Arts.

This meant I had to complete an Access to Science course before I could even set foot in a lecture theatre. I won't bore you with the details of that year, though. It was only a couple of sessions a week and I continued to work full time throughout. It was merely another hoop to jump through, another barrier between me and the printed decree of competence.

University was the usual. I had hated it for a reason the first time around and I once more struggled to see the appeal during the second attempt. Day one was done and survived, but day two was a different case of events completely. Boring was an understatement. The whole affair was unorganised, unengaging, and utterly uninspiring.

I did enjoy the 'fun' maths quiz though, mostly because I like a bit of mind-straining teamed with a little competition. I had no idea what the hell it had to do with uni induction, but I figured it might come in handy for future medication titration. Beyond that, I walked around aimlessly. I tried to fathom why I was travelling a 66-mile round trip and navigating childcare for The Boy whilst not getting paid. I was expected to trawl the extensive grounds via a quiz and map exercise that did not even have the Student's Union bar on.

All I had left to do was get through the second stage of day two. This was a three-hour social hub. The lead word says it all, and I had already rendered the process a disaster. I walked in and took a welcome pack, feeling a brief flutter of excitement at receiving a free pen. It was a blue Bic biro, not even suitable for writing nursing notes, but I clearly would not be doing that any time soon.

I quickly grasped why said free pen had been thrusted upon me. I was instantly bombarded with reps from every angle. They encouraged me to use my new redundant pen to sign up for copious amounts of "stuff," namely memberships and group subscriptions that cost a fortune. It was never quite clear what the return on investment was.

A friendly Student's Union rep approached me with incredible enthusiasm. I felt bad for not engaging with her, so I asked her the only question that came to mind. Is this event attendance based? Her excitable response was that it was not at all. She told me it was designed for me to meet, greet, and interact with my fellow cohort. I left immediately with a spring in my step and got home a bit earlier than expected. Bonus.

Day three arrived, and after a personal meltdown the night before, I woke up feeling like shit. It was one of those mornings when you realise you have been so self-absorbed by your own misery that you must acknowledge the damage. My disengagement and uncommunicative nature with the people I loved and trusted the most had led to further isolation and self-hatred.

But you must keep going. I had experience in the care sector, and I had fought to secure a place at university. Someone somewhere was looking down on me, and this possibility would only come to fruition if I was present.

I was exhausted after watching 4oD for a few hours on my mobile phone in the twilight zone of the early hours, a tactic used specifically to avoid further questioning my life choices. It was fun, however, as I watched *This Is England* and reminisced about all the questionable experiences I had. I spent my youth cajoling around with my older sisters in the nineties. They were both older than me, so I was introduced to things that perhaps I shouldn't have been at such a tender age. I still swear they are the reason for my Peter Pan-esque adult rebellion.

I had then clock-watched for what seemed like forever until a short while before my alarm was due to go off. You guessed it; I fell into a coma. After having a stern mental chat with myself and a couple of snoozes later, I remembered it was only the first few weeks of uni. It was way too soon to start throwing unauthorised absences about, so I hauled my carcass up.

The journey in was horrendous. There was a special window in the morning where a selective group of individuals found it acceptable to drive like absolute knobends. In my patch, it was those who lived out of the city and had to be at work in the centre at 09:00 yet still left their house a 08:50. They took the journey at well over the limit with copious amounts of reckless overtaking, usually in an unsuitably coloured sports car.

After throwing a few beeps of the horn and irately giving a few van drivers the universal gesture, I inevitably ran late. I was a hot mess by the time I arrived in the lecture theatre. The stress of the main roads was reverberating through my whole body as I tried to find a place to sit.

Luckily, as a result of my tardiness, I managed to bypass most social contact with my fellow cohort. I secured a seat as close to the exit as possible, providing a tactical escape route should the boredom become terminal, and awaited the joys of an introduction to Anatomy and Physiology. It was an odd start to the day, transitioning from the excitement of a road rage incident on the ring road to the dry reality of cellular biology.

That was categorically the most excited I had been thus far. I was finally getting to sit through a real-life lecture. I hoped I might come away feeling like I had learned something new, or at least finally have an indication of what was in store for the coming months. I sat back in the hard plastic chair and tried to look forward to the next few hours of my existence.

About an hour in, they finally got around to telling us the itinerary for the first A&P module. My heart sank. It was every single thing from the previous year's access course. Good god, someone, somewhere, please teach me something soon.

I desperately tried to keep positive. I told myself that at least it would be a good refresher, and since I already had a tonne of notes and books on the subject, I could probably power nap when I was bored shitless. Sitting through three-to-four-hour lectures is a brutal test of endurance. It is a slow, methodical drain on the soul that even industrial strength willpower cannot fix.

Continuing with the positive mindset, I went into manifestation mode. I decided to make a very conscious effort to actively speak to someone I had never met before whilst filtering out of the lecture theatre. That did not go to plan. Everyone already seemed to have formed small groups of a few, sticking together with fierce loyalty as if they were hunting to avoid being hunted. I decided I would try next time and hightailed it out of there at speed.

The next stage, uniform fitting. Need I say more? We were ushered into an open plan room that was nowhere near large enough for the crowd. It was full of racks upon racks of polyester that resisted the very concept of human form. It still amazes me the lengths some people will go to look good in something inherently ugly.

The upshot is simple. You will never, in your entire healthcare career be able to choose what you wear to work. Your uniform will never fit perfectly or comfortably, and you certainly won't pull in it. Or perhaps you will, but you really shouldn't. My advice is to state your size, try the bloody thing on if you absolutely have to, order it, and move on.

There is no time for intricate makeup application, elaborate hair-ups, or pouting for selfies in this environment. If you think there is, then guess what? Do not be a nurse. You are in the wrong profession. In the very near future, the most attractive adornment to your uniform will be a random person's bodily fluid. If you can't handle a boxy tunic, you certainly won't handle a stray splash of vomit.

All of my days were so similar that they merged into one. The only differential was whether I was currently at work or at university. Surprisingly, I managed to get an adequate night of sleep, but I still woke up with a sense of anguish that I knew I would have to shake off quickly. Live, die, repeat.

I treated myself to a hot bath, ensuring there was enough on the meter to justify the indulgence. I sat down with a cuppa and suddenly remembered that today was the day. Bursary and student finance payday. I logged into my online banking and stared blankly at my phone whilst the app buffered. It persisted indefinitely.

In that brief window of time, my mind was catapulting from exaltation to misery. I knew this could only go one of two ways. I was either going to be loaded or skint. The result was a bleak £8.60 in my current account. Funnily enough, there was also £2.30 of interest in my savings account, despite it having had bugger all in it for the last forever. How does that even happen? I downed my tea like it was something significantly stronger and prayed my mind had the ability to self-medicate against the impending poverty.

The hot bath did the trick and woke me up. I followed this with a moment of self-gratification as I hung my washing out at a ridiculous hour of the morning. It was a small, pathetic victory that proved I am, in actual fact, a domestic goddess. With that delusion firmly in place, I left for another day.

The journey was nowhere near as bad as the previous one. This was largely because I managed to find my old gut-wrenching, James Blunt CD, which I listened to on full whack all the way there. It was a slightly depressing choice of soundtrack, but it served a purpose. It was a reminder that misery is a competitive sport and that someone else in the world, was feeling even shittier than me.

There is a strange comfort in knowing some people legitimately make a living from writing songs about their own emotional squalor. That is exactly why I did not choose nursing as a profession. I am not here for the artistic expression of my trauma. Nursing chose me as a vocation, probably because it knew I had the stomach for the reality of it, rather than the lyrics.

I arrived safely and on time despite my mind being solely focused on the mathematics of survival. I was mentally calculating how the hell I was going to pay the rent, fill the fridge, and finance The Boy until payday. I wish I could tell you that the day was more exciting than my bank balance, but it was a slog of administrative box-ticking.

Library services followed by fire safety, followed by a three hour long break. Normal people would have used that time to socialise, but I spent it brooding. The finale was a senior student lead introduction with a specific focus on financial management. The irony was not lost on me.

The Q&A session resulted in me asking with slightly too much conviction if there was anything they could do for students who were skint, living on the breadline, and lacked the funds to even get to Uni or eat. The response was a bureaucratic shrug in verbal form. I was told I could apply for a hardship loan of up to £200. It would take a few days to approve, another couple of weeks to pay out, and required repayment in full on the first Friday of the following month.

I managed to think without verbalising the phrase: "That's a bloody no, then." It was no surprise, however, that I eventually applied for it, received it, spent it, and then promptly defaulted on the repayment. When you are drowning, a temporary lifejacket you have to pay back with interest doesn't exactly help you reach the shore.

I left feeling disheartened but bumped into a good friend from the access course. During the short walk back to our cars, she sensed the disconnect and asked if I was okay. After a long discussion that led to mutual commiseration, I expressed my frustration. I explained my disdain about how long it takes for student finance to process and admitted that I was currently living on fumes.

She did not say a word. She simply leant into her handbag, reached for her purse, and handed me forty quid. I could not formulate any words. She put her hand on my shoulder, shoved the cash into my palm, and told me to take it. She said she had been there herself and insisted it was mine.

Tears of sheer joy tinged with embarrassment flooded my eyes. Having to take a handout felt like a blow to my pride, but I thanked her through my tearful choking and headed to my car. As she headed in the opposite direction, she hollered "It's not a loan."

I climbed into my faithful car, Arryetta. She had certainly seen better days, but still functioned, mostly. I started her up and saw the fuel light was already glowing. I managed to make it to my home patch and pulled into the fuel station, but I broke down a few metres from the pump. The car would not restart. I sat there and cried.

A strapping young emergency medic happened to be there filling up. He came over to ask if I needed help and then pushed me the rest of the way to the pump. I put fuel in with the money I had been gifted and got home safely. My friend was an angel, as was the medic who abandoned their response vehicle to help me. My faith in humanity was restored. Surprisingly I was looking forward to the next day.

It dutifully arrived and I walked into the morning lecture theatre only to be faced with a few hours of SDL. It took a while to fathom out yet another one of university's million abbreviations. These acronyms seem to span and differ across all faculties and disciplines to keep us in a state of perpetual confusion.

Once the translation was complete, we all registered this meant Self Directed Learning. In plain English, it meant the session was independently self-guided and could be completed anytime and anywhere. The collective recognition hit the room like a physical wave.

We therefore all went home immediately with absolutely no intention of studying a single damn thing. If uni was going to give me the gift of time, I wasn't going to waste it on cellular biology when I had a life to piece back together and a fridge that was still suspiciously empty. I headed back to Arryetta and enjoyed the rare luxury of a morning that didn't involve a plastic chair and a PowerPoint presentation.

I arrived home super early. It was a rare, lovely afternoon spent with The Boy. With the hope of a lie-in on the horizon because the next day was only a short one, I went to bed with a genuine tinge of excitement at the prospect of not waking up to an alarm.

Unfortunately, my body clock had other ideas. I suffered through an actual nightmare involving a chaotic blur of timetables, room numbers, and placement schedules. The dream culminated in me being chased around an abandoned university grounds by lecturers dressed as clowns. It was a vivid, foreboding manifestation of my academic anxiety, and it left me very much awake at 02:10.

I decided to spend the extra time wisely. I sat in the pre-dawn quiet re-reading my timetables and studied the grounds map. I was desperately trying to work out where the hell I needed to be that afternoon and what, if anything, I was going to learn. When your brain is in survival mode, it refuses to believe that a morning off is anything other than a trap.

The Boy had a dental appointment. Since it was his first extraction, I grabbed the chance to do something motherly. It made a change from simply ferrying him to school or to the houses of family and friends to be looked after by other people. I felt like I was constantly away, studying and working for what felt like every waking hour of my life.

I initially felt like I had been a great support to him during the appointment. That feeling vanished when I had to leave him with Nanny. He had a fat face and cotton wool stuffed into his cheeks, making him resemble a hamster with big teary eyes. It made my heart hurt.

I felt that specific pain, the deep and all-consuming one that every mother feels when they wish they could take their child's suffering for them. I had another cry and told myself it was only a tooth and that I needed to get a grip. He was stabalised and supervised and I had a mandatory session to haunt.

After a long journey in through the rush hour, I arrived to discover we were meeting our academic liaisons. These are the specific people who are meant to know every finite detail of your course and your study plan. They are supposed to be the experts on when and where to get help if or when the situation requires it.

Mine was in their very first year on the job. They were a qualified nurse, so they undoubtedly knew shed loads about the clinical content of the course. However, they knew absolutely nothing about the actual course structure itself. They were adorably oblivious to the assignments, the placements, or the logistical *Hunger Games* that was our education.

I walked away from the meeting feeling none the wiser and infinitely deflated. I was still tragically unsure of what I was supposed to be studying during my SDL time. I had no idea what, if anything, I should be handing in, or even when and who I should be handing it to. It was yet another example of the blind leading the slightly more cynical blind.

There was yet more waiting. University life has a habit of putting long breaks between scheduled sessions. This might be useful if we had anything specific to study, but it is not so helpful in the first term when we don't know our arses from our elbows.

We then finally got called into the next session, which was titled PALS. This stands for Peer Assisted Learning. We sat through a brief presentation given by a few doctoral students who were all from radically different departments. Not one of them was from the clinical faculty.

None of them could answer our specific nursing-related questions. Instead, they tried with great vigour to promote the current unorganised administration. They described the chaos, which had already become a common theme amongst the cohort, as an endearing trait to studying at this particular university. You could feel the collective frustration rising in the room like a localised inflammatory response.

When they announced they were staying for another two hours to answer any questions, I decided to leave immediately. I wanted to avoid the full-scale mutiny that I was confident was about to occur. I had no interest in watching a room full of exhausted adults take their anger out on a group of confused academics who clearly didn't have any solutions apart from the standard issue "we'll find out for you.".

On my way out, I bumped into yet another friend from the previous year's foundation access course. After much encouragement, I allowed her to buy me a coffee. I literally could not afford to buy my own, let alone anyone else's. This conversation, however, did not go to plan. She informed me that when she checked in with her newly appointed academic liaison, she was notified that there had been a significant delay in university completing our enrolments.

This meant our student bursaries would not be paid until the end of the following month. This 'endearing' academic quirk was rapidly becoming an actionable offense. The thought of financial hardship to this degree for another month rendered me incapable of fighting back angry tears. My current job was just about covering my rent. I sat there with the word's food, fuel, bills circling my head, not to mention all the costs needed to support The Boy.

My friend asked what was going on and all I could blurt out was the truth about the electric. It had gone off the previous week for most of a day because I could not afford to top up the meter. As a result, I lost an entire fridge and freezer worth of food. I excused myself and went to the toilet to try and pack my uncontrollable tears into a box at the back of my head. I needed to return in a seemingly calm manner rather than appearing as a middle-aged student on the verge of a mental breakdown.

When I got back, she was gone. All that was left was a note on the table. It read that she had put something in the zip pocket of my jacket because she knew I would not take it. She said I was proud and stubborn like her. Inside was twenty-five pounds. I drove home crying with a quote I had read somewhere recently on a loop. As we grow up, we realise it is less important to have lots of friends and more important to have real ones.

University had sold us the romanticised notion that, as student nurses, we were a collective designed to nurture and sustain one another. It was a lovely, theoretical sentiment. But looking back now, I wonder exactly when the hunger set in: at what point did the pressure shift from supporting the front line to eating our own?
I had the weekend off with no shifts and a tactical decision to ignore the mountain of paperwork. It was a desperate attempt at a self-preservation mental health intervention. I knew my frequent mini meltdowns were dangerously close to becoming a permanent

16

personality trait: if I didn't schedule some genuine downtime, I would eventually be rendered unfit to be a student, let alone a nurse.

Saturday was spent with The Boy, much to his teenage disdain. I bribed his participation by driving him to a skatepark miles away to watch him assault ramps that all looked identical to the untrained eye. After an evening in an unheard-of decent night's sleep, I woke up absolutely starving. I rang The Rentals, deployed my most pathetic "starving-student-nurse-in-crisis" voice and, successfully blagged a roast dinner.

Whilst I was there, I pleaded poverty and managed to leave with half a roast chicken and a fiver. I even received a rare tap on the shoulder from a Pop's. He gave me a whisper of an admission, telling me that he was proud of what I was trying to do. I chose to ignore the word "trying" and simply took it as a win. Sundays were not so bad after all when you had a full stomach and a five pound note in your pocket.

The next day was rent day. There was still no sign of the bursary. I opened my eyes and stared blankly at the ceiling for several minutes before I remembered the small mercy of my situation. I had called the landlord and managed to get the rent delayed by a few days, and persuaded the bank to delay my direct debit.

I was incredibly lucky with my private rental. I worked at the care home where my landlord's mother resided, and she was surprisingly supportive of my academic martyrdom. While they never let me off the hook for the rent, as no one is quite *that* saintly, she didn't mind giving me some leeway. Feeling optimistic that I had successfully swerved a bank fine for non-payment, I performed a slow excavation of myself from the duvet, put the kettle on for a caffeine hit, and ran a bath to defrost my soul.

I then checked my unwanted emails and desperately avoided the book of face before consulting my timetable. Understanding that document should be a degree in itself. Then, there it was. It was that specific moment of dread that effectively ruins your entire day before it has even begun. I saw an early morning hygiene session followed by nutrition and "eat well" plates. This was to incorporate an interactive exercise of assisting patients at mealtimes via role play. Fucking role play.

The afternoon was no better. They really should have titled this lecture "An exploration into how to scare the shit out of all healthcare students." We were bombarded with assessment criteria and grading scales. If you fail a single element of anything, you are capped at a pass for the entire module. Two fails and you are out of the programme, Finished.

There is an unnegotiable perfect pass rate required for Safe Medicate by the last year. If you do not hit that perfect score, you guessed it, you are out. I could continue with the finite details of standard referencing and the tedious creation of career portfolios, but just writing this renders me with the same sick recoiling in my oesophagus as it did then.

It was the end of the week, so I went home and drowned my rising vomit in a pool of wine. It was the only logical response to such a systematic breakdown of my confidence. On the upside, however, the early morning session was surprisingly useful. We learnt how to wash our hands.

The next day I woke up a little after midnight stressing about money. Yes, I did go to bed at 20:10. I toyed with the idea of checking my banking app, but I thought better of it and decided that it was a very bad idea. I could not get back to sleep, so I changed my mind and checked it anyway. Shit me down.

The bursary was in and the student loan was in. This was the most money that had been in my bank account at any one time since my entrepreneurship days. Feeling a load lifted off my shoulders, I laid back down thinking this was going to be the best sleep I had ever experienced.

Naturally, the peace did not last. I then spent the next several hours forming a detailed mental checklist of all the bills I had to pay and the people I needed to pay back. By the time morning arrived, I had successfully spent every single penny in my head. Twice. The exaltation of being wealthy was short-lived, replaced by the grim reality of being the world's most over-qualified middleman for my own creditors.

We were finally nearing the end of the first stretch of uni. The next stop was placement. Before we could get excited about that, however, we were required to spend many hours discussing our first assignment. This was due inconveniently at the very end of the upcoming placement period.

The only premise I can assume for this timing is that the university wants to test your limits. They throw you into a clinical area for the first time, into a pack of wolves, correction, I meant Nurses. Then they add the emotional turmoil of hands-on caring for actual patients. The inclusion of a major assignment during this chaos will most probably prove your tenacity and tell you once and for all if nursing is truly for you.

If you cannot navigate that specific cocktail of stress, at least you have wasted less than a year of your life. You can pivot your entire future professional future before the debt and the trauma get too deep. It is a brutal way to filter the ranks: in the world of healthcare, the university clearly believes in survival of the most organised and the least likely to require sectioning by year three.

02

How to Be a Student Nurse and

Walk Before You Can Run

If you are anything like me, you entered nursing with a dangerous level of delusion. I expected urgency. I expected trauma. I expected to be saving lives before my morning coffee. Instead, I was trapped in a windowless lecture theatre. The topic was "Communication." Again. The cohort sat in a vegetative state, enduring learning outcomes we had covered for a thousand hours. Then the rumbling started. It spread like a contagion. The tutor faltered, confused by the sudden shift from coma to riot. Placements were live. The whispering escalated into full-volume panic and a healthy smattering of profanity. The cohort was revolting. Above the din, I heard the screams of the damned.

"I can't travel that far!"

"How am I supposed to get there for six?"

"Gastro? Is that shit? That's definitely shit."

I sat there, absorbing the misery. I felt a smug sense of superiority. I silently contemplated, you knew what you signed up for. Suck it up. Then my phone pinged. Rehabilitation. "For fuck's sake." So much for the moral high ground.

The truth was, nursing was rarely like *Casualty*. Most avenues didn't involve emergency sirens or open-heart surgery in a lift. It was holistic. It was person-centred. It was mostly about stopping people dying from boredom or neglect.

You learnt something everywhere, even if it was where not to work. I dragged my heels into placements I expected to loathe and left heartbroken. Conversely, I walked into others expecting to find my calling and left knowing I would rather scrub toilets than work there.

Rehabilitation was a relatively modern invention. The first hospital reportedly opened in Brinley in 1998. It was designed as a halfway house for patients who were medically fit for discharge but would likely accidentally kill themselves if sent home alone. It prevented readmission and reduced "delayed discharges": the polite term for bed blocking.

I was sent to a local community hospital with twenty beds. It had since been closed, thanks to a misguided decision by the regional authority. These vital "restoration" services were being scrapped because the government claimed they weren't financially viable. Apparently, "care at home" was cheaper, even if the patient was mostly alone and terrified.

That was only my opinion. I urged you to research the politics of your placement. It gives you excellent substance for your Quality Improvement assignment. This is a soul-destroying piece of coursework that coincided with your Literature Review.

Day one started surprisingly well. I met the team and my mentor. These units ran on a specific fuel mix: nurses, physios, OTs, and social workers, all trying to get the patient fit enough to leave. The hierarchy was clear. Senior Charge Nurses, Advanced Clinical Practitioners, and the formidable Modern Matron. Unlike acute wards, this wasn't doctor-led. We relied on primary care clinicians. If things got complicated, we called the cavalry: Speech and Language, Dietitians, or Psychological Support.

A quick word of advice for a placement such as this is: use your "Spokes."

Your placement is the hub; spokes are short visits to specialist areas. They were priority passes to see things your general placement won't cover. But they wouldn't come to you. You had to hustle. You needed to sell yourself with knowledge and enthusiasm. Even in nursing, it isn't always what you know, but who you impress.

Introductions over, my mentor decided I needed grounding. I was assigned to shadow the Healthcare Assistants.

I felt a pang of disappointment. I wasn't "too posh to wash", I'd spent years in the trenches as a care assistant myself, but I was desperate to get my hands on the nursing work. I wanted drug rounds, not bed baths. Still, I smiled. I am a firm believer in leading from the front. If you aren't prepared to wipe an arse, you have no business administering the laxatives.

I was paired with Rae. She had been there six months. Rae explained she had been long-term unemployed until the Jobcentre found them an "entry to healthcare" course. I nodded, wholly impressed. I loved a good underdog story. I asked if she had enjoyed the training, expecting a heartwarming tale of vocational discovery. Rae looked at me with dead eyes. "No. I hated it. It was fucking boring and I don't like old people." I blinked. "Right. So why did you take the job?" "Coz they said they'd cut my benefits otherwise." Ah. The Florence Nightingale spirit lives on.

Rae took their instructions to "train me" very literally. I was informed that I was to watch, observe, and under no circumstances touch anything or anyone. I was essentially a potted plant with a uniform. We entered the first room. I stepped forward to introduce myself, but Rae cut me off with a wave of her hand. She turned to the patient. "Don't worry about her. She's just a student. I'm going to show her how we do our job."

If this hadn't been Day One and I wasn't "just a student" I would have marched her into the sluice room and given her a masterclass in patient care. Instead, I swallowed the rage. There is a lot to be said for first impressions, even if that impression is of someone grinding their teeth into dust.

By patient number four, it was blindingly obvious. To Rae, these weren't people. They were objects. They were tasks on a to-do list to be scrubbed and ticked off. There was no dignity. There was no conversation. There was no compassion. Then came the last straw.

I followed Rae into the next room. Meet Mara. They had recently been admitted post-stroke with dense left-sided weakness and significant aphasia. Rae didn't waste time on pleasantries. She began undressing Mara with the grace of a mechanic stripping an engine. She became distressed immediately. I moved to the bedside. I calmly asked if they would mind if I sat in their armchair. She looked at me with an intensity that was almost painful. Tears pooled in her eyes. They nodded towards the chair. Rae was disgruntled. She ushered me into the ensuite. In a voice that was supposed to be a whisper but sounded like a foghorn, she told me to "observe only." I kept my voice level. "If I talk to them, it might reduce their anxiety. They will be more compliant." Rae rolled her eyes. "Whatever. As long as I get done quicker."

I went back to Mara. I talked them through every movement, pre-empting Rae's rough handling. Mara calmed almost immediately. Then it was time to get dressed. While Rae was busy, I went to the wardrobe. I offered Mara a choice from a small, ill-fitting selection. She pointed to a pretty long-sleeved jumper. Rae snatched the garment from my hand and mumbled, "I'm never going to get that on them." She proceeded to shove Mara's strong arm in first. Then yanked it over her head like a wet shroud from a cadaver. Finally, she tried to forcibly wedge the dead-weight left arm into the remaining sleeve. It was like watching someone try to put a wetsuit on a cat. I couldn't take it anymore.

"Rae. May I?" She stared at me incredulously. "If I can't do it, you're not going to be able to." I removed the jumper. I turned to Rae. "If you do the weak arm first, then the head, Mara can do the rest herself." Rae scoffed. "Yeah, right." I ignored them. I turned to the patient. "Mara, shall we try that again? I'm here if you need help." With a nod, I guided the weak arm in. Then gently placed over her head. Mara used her strong arm to pull it down and adjust the waist. She was dressed. We walked out into the corridor. Rae looked at me with the intensity of a landlady about to call time. "Does that trick work every time?" "Pretty much," I replied. "Where did you learn that?" I smiled sweetly. "During the six years I worked as a care assistant before I started my nurse training." Safe to say, Rae's attitude performed a screeching U-turn.

After a few days of proving I wasn't useless, it was time to shadow my mentor. First up: the drug round. My mentor was a veteran. She had over thirty years of service under her belt. She was proper Old School. She was the type of nurse who commanded respect without opening her mouth. When she walked onto the ward, spines straightened. The radio was turned down. You did not use her first name. She was Nurse Calder. God help you if you forgot it.

Rehabilitation units were a clinical tombola. They threw every eventuality and co-morbidity at you. One minute you were helping a post-fracture patient mobilise down the corridor. The next, you were titrating oxygen for a gasping COPD patient. You were dressing surgical wounds. You were managing PEG feeds. And that was the highlights reel. You saw everything there. You treated it all.
As a care assistant, I had witnessed plenty of drug rounds. I had even assisted the Nurse in Charge under strict supervision. I thought I knew

the drill. I was wrong. I hadn't anticipated the sheer logistical nightmare of medicating twenty people. I say twenty because, while the official ratio was a safe one-to-ten, staff sickness usually turned that into a daunting one-to-twenty.

Technically, there was always a Band 6 on shift. Theoretically, she was there to help. In reality she was usually buried under a mountain of admission paperwork and discharge planning. She was too busy fighting a losing battle against the clock to rescue me.

And so, the trolley rolled. Medication rounds were routinely performed at breakfast, lunch, evening, and night. That sounded manageable. It wasn't. You also had to factor in the outliers. There were the early morning doses. The pre-food doses. The post-food doses. Then there were the time-critical terrors: Parkinson's meds, insulin, anti-seizure prescriptions and the list goes on like a never-ending shopping list for a chemist that has already run out of stock. You needed your wits about you. You needed to know your patient's routine better than your own. You had to stay on the ball because a missed dose wasn't a minor inconvenience. It caused detrimental physical effects for the patient. It also led to the dreaded "Medication Error." When you qualified, you were solely responsible. You were wholly accountable. Buckle up. In this job, there is zero room for error.

Nurse Calder was a rain man of pharmaceuticals. She knew every single Medication Administration Record off by heart. She glided between patients with high-octane precision, never missing a beat. She laid out the battle plan. "We go to rooms 2, 11, and 16 first. They need pre-breakfast meds. Then we loop back and do the routine run from room 1 to 20. Once they are done, we circle back for the timed medications. Finally, we move to the two patients who need their PEG feeds hung." I frantically tried to scribble this tactical manoeuvre into my pocket notepad. I soon gave up. I decided to rely on observation and prayer. I hoped my memory didn't file for divorce. True to form, Nurse Calder treated the drug round like a sadistic game show.

"Victoria, indication for Bisoprolol?"

"Pre-administration check for Digoxin?"

"Blood glucose is 18. Do we give the insulin?"

Did I know the answers? Some. All of them? Definitely not.

The public shaming worked. It encouraged me to learn every single drug I touched. I became obsessive. I catalogued empty packets. I filed Patient Information Leaflets. I studied the Formulary until my eyes bled. My fellow student on placement ridiculed me. I let her laugh. We didn't realise then that university provided very little actual pharmacology training. You got the odd dry lecture on the chemical makeup of ACE Inhibitors or Beta Blockers, but zero instruction on brand names or dosage. Instead, uni offered "Safe Medicate." It was an online programme. It taught you the maths. It taught you how to calculate a volume. It did not teach you what the drug was primarily used for, or how to avoid killing a patient with it. You were required to sit a Safe Medicate exam every year. The pass mark climbed steadily. By year three, you needed 100%. You only got two attempts. Yes. I said 100%.

***

Have you ever heard the phrase "making a mountain out of a molehill"? Well, here came my molehill. And I was about to die on it. After four weeks of shadowing Nurse Calder, I was essentially a highly qualified voyeur. I had observed everything. Drug rounds, wound dressings, catheter care, care planning. It was educational, but I was beginning to feel like a broken infusion pump. I tentatively asked if I

26

could do something. I wanted to get my hands dirty under supervision. Nurse Calder shut me down. "Your role is to observe. You must work within your competency."

I gritted my teeth. It was the ultimate nursing Catch-22. How exactly did one improve competency without ever being allowed to demonstrate ability? I was stuck in a loop. My Practice Assessment Portfolio remained dangerously blank. It was very easy to go with the flow. It was safer to do as you were told. But I warn you: a placement is only twelve weeks long. You might have thought that sounded like an eternity. Believe me, it flies by faster than a rumour on a night shift.

I tried gentle persuasion. It was like talking to a brick wall. I was hit with the standard playlist of excuses.

"I'm not sure you're ready."

"Time is against us today."

"Perhaps if you wrote me an essay on the theoretical underpinnings first."

My frustration was climbing the walls. I decided to force the issue and request a formal meeting. For the uninitiated, placements required four mandatory interviews: Orientation, Preliminary, Formative, and Summative. These were the evidence base for your grading. Without them, you failed.

Nurse Calder agreed, but with caveats. We could meet only if every single clinical task was finished to her satisfaction. Alternatively, she graciously offered for me to come in on my day off to discuss my "concerns" while she was on shift. My day off? If she was on shift, how would that magically manufacture the time to speak to me?

Confused and disappointed, I backed down. I waited for a gap in the clouds that never came.

We finally managed to sit down. The discussion was very much led by me. I went straight for the jugular: when would I be considered ready to formally partake in the job I was breaking my back to learn for a bursary that was less living wage and more contribution to my eventual liver failure. The responses were pure waffle. There was no substance. "You are keen," she said, "but you tend to rush. You should take a step back." It felt like a criticism. It probably was. But then, Nurse Calder did something I never expected. She flipped the script. The iron lady began to question her own abilities. Was she teaching me enough? Was I pleased with her training style? Had I learnt anything from her? I was floored by this sudden vacuum of confidence. The meeting concluded with me reassuring her. It was a farce. As a result of this bizarre therapy session, Nurse Calder arranged for me to meet the Modern Matron. Brilliant.

Next shift, a miracle occurred. We were fully staffed. Nurse Calder let me take the reins on the morning medication round. I was in my element, dispensing pills under her hawk-like supervision. Then the Junior Charge Nurse strolled over. I was summoned to the manager's office to meet the Modern Matron. The walk was only a few metres, but it felt like the Green Mile. I had zero time to prepare a defence. I tried to arrange my grievances into a diplomatic bouquet, omitting any direct blame. I knocked. The Matron waved me in and gestured for me to sit. She didn't speak. She flicked through my Practice Assessment Portfolio and a stack of handwritten notes like a bailiff looking for the one thing in the house worth seizing.'

My hands went clammy. My heart took up a frantic, hollow percussion against my sternum. God, what have I done? I should have kept my head down and my mouth shut. (You will hear that mantra a lot in this game). Finally, she spoke. "So, Victoria. How have you been getting

28

on?" I decided on tactical flattery. I commended the team. I lied about how much I was enjoying the "learning process." The Matron looked up. "Well, where are we going wrong then?" The question hit me like a freight train. I dropped the act. "I feel ready to begin demonstrating my knowledge. I need to be proactive with treatments, not just watch them." She paused. It was an uncomfortable, heavy silence that lasted a lifetime. She flicked through another page. "I agree. I'll speak with Nurse Calder. This needs to be fixed. We need to do better." Whether "we" meant the unit, or "we" meant Nurse Calder, I wasn't sure. But the effect was instant. By the end of the following week, the floodgates opened. I had completed all daily medication rounds, redressed bilateral leg ulcers, packed a surgical wound, titrated an insulin infusion, and managed a rapidly deteriorating patient without killing them. I was finally a student nurse.

***

Next up: Occupational Therapy. Our lead OT was Morgan. He visited three times a week to perform miracles, or at least to install grab rails. Their remit was vast. An OT assessment is the gatekeeper of discharge. Working in tandem with the sadists in Physiotherapy, they review the patient. They construct a treatment plan. They produce a comprehensive risk assessment. The goal is simple: ensure the patient can return to their own home without immediately breaking a hip and bouncing straight back to us.

It wasn't only about the patient; it was about the habitat. Was the home fit for purpose? Or was it a death trap of loose rugs and steep stairs? I found myself weirdly drawn to the logistics of a safe discharge. Whenever I had a spare minute, I pestered Morgan about the minutiae of their day. We bonded over a shared, pathological need to cross every 't' and dot every 'i'. We were kindred spirits in bureaucracy. It wasn't long before they invited me to shadow them on a day of house calls and environmental assessments. This was a Type O-negative moment. It was the only time I didn't have to beg, borrow, or steal to get a Spoke placement. With the blessing of Nurse Calder and university, I jumped at the chance. I was going to be an OT for the day.

What an eye-opener. That day shed a harsh light on the NHS. It wasn't just about medicine; it was a crash course in the complexities of administration and the crushing impact of politics. Everything I thought I knew was thrown into the incinerator. We bounced between two different worlds.

First, we visited a freezing country cottage built for Minpins; where trying to manoeuvre a standard issue walking frame was like trying to parallel park an articulated lorry in a walk-in wardrobe. The occupants were living in complete poverty, struggling to heat the single room they lived in. The elderly wife was waiting for her husband to return from the hospital. Despite the cold, she declined all assistance. She refused the care package. She was fiercely, painfully independent. "I care for him. It's my duty. We don't need anybody coming in and disturbing us. We will be fine." We left her to her pride and drove to "The Estate."

The contrast was enough to give you whiplash. This place had actual staff who summoned the patient's son. He was wearing a tailored suit, a silk cravat, and a matching pocket square. He didn't offer us a cup of tea. Instead, he demanded a stairlift to cover all three floors. He specifically requested it be colour-coordinated with the décor. He also requested a live-in Service nurse. He wasn't sure "Mummy" would be safe with just the housemaid looking in on her. The poor ask for nothing. The rich ask for everything.

***

My placement was nearing its end. It was time for the closure review and the completion of the dreaded Practice Assessment Portfolio.

Given my rocky start, the mountain of written reflections, and the regular summons to the Matron's office, I was feeling nothing short of intense panic. It was pure, unadulterated fear. What if I'd failed? What if I had to repeat? What if my journey was over before I'd even bought my first fob watch?

The fear was justified. Rumours were already circulating about a student who had been removed halfway through the placement. They had been stationed in a secure mental health unit. In a moment of madness, they approached a patient unsupervised and asked them to recount their past traumas in extreme detail. They claimed their intention was "healing," drawn from their own personal struggles. They thought it would be therapeutic. I am not sure if they meant for them or the patient. The result was catastrophic. The patient spiralled and self-harmed. Needless to say, the student was shoved out of the exit. They work in IT now. At least computers don't bleed when you ask them the wrong questions.

I still don't know if I winged it. Perhaps I survived through sheer bloody-mindedness. Maybe, just maybe, I did a good job. The verdict was in. I passed. I didn't scrape a pass. I scored 98 out of 100. That put me in the 88th percentile. It turns out that challenging your colleagues is sometimes appreciated, provided you do it professionally. It is a risky game, but sometimes having a backbone pays off. Not with everyone, obviously. But with some.

The glow of the ninety-eight lasted exactly ten minutes. Then the neurosis set in. Which questions did I fail? I started a forensic audit of my Practice Assessment Portfolio. If I could score ninety-eight, surely I could score a hundred? I scanned the twenty criteria. I correlated the scores. It didn't make any sense. I had only dropped a single mark on Question 17: 'Takes appropriate responsibility for any difficulties encountered.' I did the maths. I did it again. If I only dropped one mark, I had scored ninety-nine. Nurse Calder had written ninety-eight. It was only one point. But it was my point.

I wrestled with myself. Should I leave it? Would challenging the score make me look ungrateful? Was I being a malcontent, checking a miracle for its expiry date? But the hunger for that clean sweep was gnawing at me. If I didn't ask, how would I fix Question 17 for next time?

I decided on a tactical approach. I wouldn't mention the bad maths. Instead, I would frame it as a hunger for self-improvement. "Nurse Calder, I would welcome some feedback on Question 17. I want to ensure I can develop in the future." The approach worked. She smiled. And, boy, am I glad I plucked up the courage to ask. You would not believe the discussion that came next. "Victoria, you don't need to improve at all. Keep doing what you are doing." She sighed, the weariness of thirty years in the national health machine washing over her.

"The only reason I didn't give you 100 is because it triggers moderation. If I give a perfect score, I must sit through yet another unpaid advanced mentorship training course. I don't have the time. You would have got 100 otherwise." She pointed to the bottom of the sheet. "Oh, and look at point 20. Valued and respected team member. I gave you a 5+ because I can't mark over 5." I stood there. Baffled, but stoked. I took the win.

I contemplated Nurse Calder's response. I tried to let it go, but I couldn't help myself. I had to get to the bottom of it. Out came the Practice Assessment Portfolio. I started reading the mundane small print, the procedural waffle I usually ignored. And there it was. Staring at me in black and white. See below, verbatim.

"PLEASE NOTE: Following submission, Practice Assessment is subject to a review process. This will involve review of the process of assessment, marks awarded and evidence/commentary documented to ensure parity wherever possible.

Where there are any queries that arise, mentors may be contacted by their academic liaison prior to final confirmation of the marks awarded. Students achieving overall marks of below 45 and above 85 will be subject to the review process".

I read it. Then re-read it. Then I stared at the wall. So, mediocrity was safe, but excellence triggered an audit? I was effectively being penalised for doing well. I now had to justify why I had scored so high. The only printable word for it was ludicrous.

Sadly, this backwards logic became an unwelcome theme. You will hear plenty more about it on this journey.

My last day was deceptive. It started as a standard shift. Then after the lunchtime drug round, the Modern Matron summoned my fellow student and me to the meeting room. She called it a "debrief." We exchanged looks of sheer terror and marched to our doom. We opened the door. "Surprise!" It was a leaving party. The room was packed with the team and every mobile patient. Even the elusive MDT members had paused their rounds to pop in. There were balloons. There were cards. Best of all, there was cake. An obscene amount of cake.

I was floored. "Overwhelmed" is an understatement. I had been so focused on the work, the training, and the bureaucracy, that I hadn't noticed the shift. In this job, you trauma-bond quickly. In twelve short weeks, these colleagues had become friends. Some of them remain so to this day.

We worked the room. We thanked everyone who had abandoned their patients to say goodbye. There were the usual pleasantries about "don't be a stranger" and the vague promises of a job once we qualified. The highlight was Nurse Calder. She made an actual speech. She announced that not only had we been sterling students, but we had taught them to be better mentors. Even the Modern Matron claimed she was proud to host us rookies.

Then came the curveball. Rae. The person who hated "old people" told me they would miss me. They thanked me for the lessons. They even announced they were enrolling in their Level 3 care qualification to get better at the job. I took that as a massive win. Maybe I will make it as a Nurse after all?

Looking back, this was a fantastic experience. It was a highlight of my training, despite the hiccups. But I must warn you. Not every placement is this idyllic. As you were about to find out, some were a very different beast entirely.

03

How to Be a Student Nurse and

Your Loan Is Not Your Income

Placement one was in the bag. I hadn't just survived; I had banked a score of ninety-eight percent, absolute proof that the agony of leaving The Boy every morning was yielding a return. I walked away with a glowing reference and a few new numbers in my phone from nurses I would trust with my life, or at least with my airway.

Even the conflict with my placement supervisors had been sanded down into something resembling mutual respect. I had treated the ward like a battlefield and won, but the victory lap was short. The uniform went into the wash, the lanyard went into the drawer, and I was dragged back to the lecture theatre. The twelve-week rotation was supposed to offer a balanced diet of theory and practice; mostly, it offered whiplash.

To the average undergraduate, a university block was a time for reading, drinking, and perhaps a little light expanding of the mind. To me, it was a logistical gap that needed to be plugged with paid work. The schedule was technically three or four days on campus a week, with the rest designated as "self-directed study." In academic terms, this meant reading journals in the library. In my terms, it meant wrestling into a tunic and working fifty hours a week as a care assistant to stop the bailiffs from taking an interest in the front door.

There were, of course, optional extras. Guest lecturers, student societies, and extracurricular bonding exercises designed to enrich the soul. You can probably guess how many of those I attended. While my cohort was busy padding their CVs or joining the ultimate frisbee team, I was busy changing incontinence pads for minimum wage.

It was back-breaking, soul-grinding work, but every hour clocked was a singular act of sabotage against poverty. It meant The Boy had school shoes. It meant the fridge hummed with actual food inside it. Most importantly, it was a war chest. I knew the next clinical placement was coming, which meant twelve weeks of working for free. I had to earn enough now to survive the drought later.

The downside to this academic purgatory was the geography. The commute was a vampire attached to my bank account, sucking away petrol money I didn't have. Worse still were the gaps in the timetable. I spent hours sitting in the canteen, guarding a table I hadn't bought anything for, unable to afford even a biscuit, staring at a textbook just to avoid eye contact with the staff.

I quickly recognised that a hair-raising percentage of nurse training had absolutely nothing to do with keeping people alive. I wanted anatomy, physiology, pharmacology; the mechanics of how to fix a broken body. Instead, we got endless modules on 'Compassion,' 'Kindness,' 'Respect' and a Code of Conduct that render you professionally lobotomised.

I said it then, and I would carve it into the desk now: compassion was not an academic subject. It could not be taught via PowerPoint or awkward role-play scenarios where one student pretended to be a dying grandmother and the other pretended to care. If you needed a university tutor to explain to you what empathy was, or a workshop to teach you that sick people deserved kindness, you were in the wrong building. Put the uniform down, walk out the door, and go work in Finance. The spreadsheets wouldn't mind that you had a heart of stone, but the patients certainly would.

I scanned the module list for the next couple of years and felt a cold drop of sweat slide down my spine. The university seemed intent on training me to be a professional hand-holder, but I was already an expert in that field. I could de-escalate a confused dementia patient or comfort a grieving relative in my sleep. What I couldn't do, and what the curriculum seemed in no rush to teach me, was how survive in a high-tech acute ward. I could count on one hand the number of times I had set foot inside a hospital. I was about to be qualified to work in a major teaching hospital, a place of revolutionary surgeries and cutting-edge trauma care, and my entire clinical experience consisted of tea, toast, and toileting.

I made a decision. It was time to sabotage my sanity for experience. I decided to quit my job.

When I told my parents, they looked at me as if I had announced I was joining a cult. To be fair, their concern was valid. At the time, I was working in a care home that was literally attached to my flat. My commute involved opening the front door and walking a few paces. I shared a party wall with the residents; I could practically tap out a conversation in Morse code with the old lady in Room 6 while I was watching *EastEnders*.

This arrangement was a single mother's dream. I could finish a twelve-hour shift and be showered, fed, and unconscious before my colleagues had even started their cars. It also meant The Boy could be left "home alone" in a legally grey but practically safe capacity. If he needed me, he didn't even need a phone; all he had to do was bang on the living room wall. Giving that up wasn't just ambitious. It was logistical suicide.

Once the gears in my head ground into position, there was no reverse. I didn't do "sleeping on it." I didn't do "pros and cons lists." I simply identified the target and walked through whatever walls were in the way. I needed to be in that major hospital. I needed to understand the hierarchy from the bottom up. I wanted to know exactly what a care assistant faced on a twelve-hour shift in Acute Medical, not only to build my own skills, but so that one day, when I was the one wearing the blue tunic, I would know exactly what I was asking of my team. The major hospital didn't recruit individuals; it harvested them. They ran massive "recruitment drives," a term that summons images of cattle being herded into a pen. The process involved submitting a forest's worth of paperwork. I provided enough documentation to satisfy a border control agent, followed by endless weeks of silence, then a flurry of interviews. The logic of the role was simple: they hired a pool of bodies and deployed us wherever the staffing crisis was currently bleeding out the fastest.

After a couple of months of waiting and a few weeks of administrative hoop-jumping, I received the hall pass. I was in. There was one final hurdle: a mandatory, full-time, two-week induction programme. I was ready. I was keen. I was also a catastrophic liability. I had assumed, like a rational person living in the twenty-first century, that labour was exchanged for currency. I should have checked the fine print. The induction was unpaid. I was about to spend two weeks burning diesel and paying for childcare, and the national health machine wasn't going to give me a penny for the privilege.

Despite the lack of a pay check, the training was the first time I felt like I was learning a trade rather than reading about one. It was a damning indictment of the higher education system that I learned more clinically in two weeks of unpaid labour than I had in sixteen months of university tuition. I became fluent in the language of survival: National Early Warning Scores, the subtle grey pallor of a deteriorating patient, and the rhythmic violence of BLS.

The fear began to evaporate. I learned to stand in a high-pressure environment without wanting to bolt for the fire exit. I could finally speak to consultants, those deities with stethoscopes, without stuttering or breaking out in hives. It clicked. They were mechanics, and I was learning how to hand them the wrench.

The major hospital was a complex assembly plant compared to the care home. The care home had soft edges, boiled cabbage, and slow decline. The major hospital was sharp, metallic, and smelled of chlorine and electricity. It was a machine. A colossal, monstrous engine of cogs and pistons. On good days, it hummed with perfect synchronicity, processing human bodies like a high-end factory. On bad days, it was a broken hunk of metal, grinding gears and chewing people up. Every morning, I walked through the sliding doors, I had to guess which version of the machine I was walking into.

There must have been a specific law of physics that dictated the moment you attempted to improve your situation in life, the universe would immediately throw a brick at your head. It was the kind of obstacle designed to make you question your sanity, forcing you to lie awake at 3 a.m. wondering if you should have stayed in your lane. I could have stuck to the original plan. I could have stayed in the care home, wrapped in the cotton wool of the care pathway, safe in the knowledge that I was competent and comfortable.

But I was incapable of settling. Whether it was delusion, hope, or a pathological inability to sit still, I could not accept that "just about managing" was the peak of human existence. I was convinced that leaving my safe, warm, easy job was the pathway to fulfilment. I was right, in theory. In practice, I was about to be punished for my hubris.

The punishment came in the form of mechanical failure. My car didn't feign break down; it died. It suffered a catastrophic, terminal event.

Suddenly, the geography of my life collapsed. I had traded a job where my commute was shorter than the time it takes to boil a kettle for a position at a major hospital on the dark side of the county. I had abandoned the managers who nurtured me for a corporate monolith, assuming my car would be the one reliable gear in my new life. Now I was stranded in the equivalent of the English outback, a lawless land where public transport was a rumour rather than a service. I was trying to secure a Bachelor of Science and work twelve-hour shifts, and I was now at the mercy of a bus timetable that seemed to have been written by someone who had never even left the town.

This was the point in the disaster movie where the family was supposed to rally. My family dynamic was complicated; my sister and I had a relationship that would require a separate memoir and a team of psychiatrists to unpack. Suffice it to say, she viewed my crisis with deep suspicion. Her husband, however, was a different breed. He was one of those useful men who owned tools and knew how to actually use them. A true fixer. While I was hyperventilating about bus timetables, he went into problem-solving mode.

He found me a car. He didn't just find four wheels and an engine; he found a vehicle that passed a vetting process I didn't have the mental capacity to understand. I buy cars based on colour and hope. He bought cars based on service history, inspection records, and a forensic check for outstanding finance. He ensured I wasn't buying a "cut and shut", which was essentially two crashed cars welded together in a shed. That was exactly the sort of death trap I would have accidentally purchased on my own.

He had found the perfect solution. It was reliable, safe, and available immediately. There was one small, unsettling snag. The price tag was three thousand eight hundred pounds. And I needed to find it. Fast. I found a lifeline on a university noticeboard. It was a private company offering "hardship loans" for students in full-time education. Usually, when something looked too good to be true, it was because there was a shark swimming just beneath the surface. But desperation quieted the survival instinct, so I applied.

The process was less like a loan application and more like a forensic autopsy of my lack of financial stability. They demanded a mountain of evidence: proof of income, proof of outgoings, and a few months of bank statements. They scrutinised every penny I spent. I had to justify why I bought a coffee on a Tuesday or why my grocery bill was higher in winter. It was humiliating, invasive, and necessary.

I am telling you this because you need to understand the odds. Securing a loan as a mature student was hard. Securing three thousand eight hundred pounds as a single mother with a credit history that looked like a crime scene was impossible. My credit file still bore the scars of my "play days," a period of youthful financial idiocy that ensured computer algorithms automatically rejected me. I was a walking red flag to lenders. Yet, opposed to all logic and risk assessment protocols, they said yes.

The 3 a.m. panic attacks returned. These weren't the gentle insomnias of a restless mind; they were full-blown, sheet-drenching terrors where you woke up with a pulse rate that would trigger a crash call on an acute ward. I was technically one of the lucky ones. My cohort was the last to receive the national bursary, the final group of students to be trained for free before the government decided that the privilege of choosing the fundamentals of care as a career should come with a north of thirty-thousand-pound price tag. I look at students after me, saddled with tuition debt before they'd even qualified, and I want to weep for them.

But even with the bursary, the financial tightrope was razor thin. Because I worked to feed The Boy, the system decided I was "earning too much" to qualify for extra support. It was a special kind of systemic irony to tell a single mother on minimum wage that she was too wealthy for assistance. I had to work to survive, but working penalised me. The new loan for the car had saved my logistics but ruined my blood pressure. I was a whisper under four grand in the hole, driving a car I couldn't afford to fix, to a job I couldn't afford to quit. I had to get a grip on the panic.

Getting my anxiety under control would have been a lovely ambition, but the university had other plans. As my heart rate was returning to double digits, the results for our first assignment landed in my inbox. This was the essay they had sadistically set during our first placement, designed to test our mettle while we were already exhausted. I clicked the link. I scanned for the number. I had passed. But it wasn't a victory; it was a near-miss. I had scraped through by exactly three marks.

I stared at the screen. I was not used to mediocrity. I had scored ninety-eight percent in clinical practice; I was practically Saint Bernadette reborn on the ward. Yet here, in the world of academic referencing and critical analysis, I was apparently a few points away from being a failure. It stopped me dead in my tracks. A pass was technically a pass, just as a car crash you walk away from was technically a successful journey. It just didn't feel like one. I had survived, but I was bleeding. I needed to know why.

The results landed on everyone's phones simultaneously, like a Pavlovian bell triggering mass hysteria. I looked up to see a sea of smiling faces and high-fives. The room erupted into the squeals of people who had validated their own intelligence. I felt the cold, familiar nausea of the school playground wash over me. I needed to evacuate.

The questions started firing like tracer rounds. "What did you get?" "Did you pass?" "I got seventy-two percent, what about you?"

I didn't answer. I tactically withdrew. I fled the building before I had to admit that, according to the university grading matrix, I was barely literate. I retreated to the safety of my car, harbouring a cocktail of embarrassment and disgust. I had prevented patients dying on the ward, but apparently, I couldn't write an essay to save my own skin.

In the sanctuary of my not new but new to me vehicle, I opened my laptop. I was hurt, but mostly I was furious. I drafted an email to my academic advisor. In hindsight, it was a message that could have benefited from a twenty-four-hour cooling-off period and a heavy edit. Instead, it was raw, defensive, and accusatory.

Let this be a lesson to anyone reading: never hit "send" when your heart rate is high enough to trigger an alarm on a cardiac monitor. Electronic communication was forever, and rage was a terrible editor.

I eventually summoned the courage to read the feedback without throwing the laptop out of the window. The diagnosis was clear. It turns out I have a talent for exams and a decent grasp of the English language, but I suffered from a fatal flaw: I had an opinion.

In the world of nursing academia, your thoughts are irrelevant. The markers do not care what you think about patient safety; they care what Author et al. (1945) thinks about patient safety. I had filled my essay with independent thought and critical analysis. This was a rookie mistake. The sooner you realise that your personal perspective is unwelcome, the sooner your grades will improve.

I had naively assumed that my previous victories, namely the GCSEs, the A Levels, and the Distinction in my Access to Health Science course, had prepared me for this. I thought I knew how to write. I thought I knew how to construct an argument. Did I bollocks. I was playing draughts, and the university was playing three-dimensional chess with a rulebook written in Latin.

The feedback sheet read like it had been written by a robot designed to suck the joy out of the English language. It demanded a "sophisticated blending of theoretical knowledge and practical application," a phrase that sounds less like nursing and more like the instructions for a high-end food processor. It lectured me on "unwavering adherence to

43

professional standards" and the holy grail of all nursing essays, "grounding your work in Evidence-Based Practice."

Then came the heavy hitters. The professional regulator's Code was invoked like a religious text. I was told I lacked "critical analysis," "reflection," and "adherence to academic conventions." Typing those words out now triggers a kinetic response. I could feel the gastric reflux starting. It wasn't feedback; it was an assassination of my writing style using a dictionary of buzzwords as the weapon. The message was clear. They didn't want a nurse who could write; they wanted an academic who could reference.

I sat there wondering if I had suffered a neurological episode during the first few weeks of term. I had attended every lecture, yet I couldn't recall a single session that explained these mystical academic requirements in any useful detail. Unless the module on "How To Not Write Like a Human Being" was held at 4 a.m. in a basement I didn't know about, as far as I was concerned, they hadn't taught it.

The only comfort came when we were herded back into the main lecture theatre. These rooms were designed to amplify sound, so when one brave soul at the back whispered that they had failed, the confession travelled like a contagion. It wasn't Chinese whispers; it was an epidemic of truth.

The cliques began to fracture. The bravado evaporated. Row by row, the admissions started tumbling out. I wasn't the village idiot; I was part of a village of idiots. Even one of my closest friends broke. They had lied to my face earlier, claiming a solid pass, but as the room descended into collective misery, they crumbled. They admitted they had failed and were in a state of total meltdown, secretly pulling all-nighters to rewrite their submission while terrified of being found out. It probably didn't uphold the professional Code regarding honesty, but it certainly upheld the human instinct for self-preservation.

It forced us to ask the question: was the university simply incompetent at teaching us, or was this deliberate? Perhaps failing half the cohort on the first hurdle wasn't an accident. Maybe it was another form of triage. Sink or swim.

I swallowed the bile, closed the email and opened my submitted assignment. I stopped self-indulging and started dissecting the feedback like a forensic pathology report. If they wanted "unwavering adherence to professional standards," I would give them so much they would choke on it.

By this point, the actual subject matter was irrelevant. "Effective communication" was the furthest thing from my mind; I was communicating purely to appease the academic gods. I would have happily written ten thousand words on the mating habits of dust mites if it meant getting a distinction.

I decided to take a gamble. Most institutions offered a form of academic Russian Roulette: the voluntary resubmission. It came with a health warning. If you had already passed, even by the skin of your teeth, and you chose to resubmit to chase a higher grade, the new grade was final. If you rewrote it and made it worse, you were stuck with the lower score. You could not go back to your original safety net.

I looked at my borderline pass. I looked at the blank page. I took the shot. I reworked every sentence until it was dripping with references and devoid of personality. The result? I shot up to the eighty-eighth percentile. It was a massive victory, but let's be clear: if I had scored that the first time around, I would have taken the win, closed the laptop, never looking back at the document again. Perfectionism is a luxury; survival is mandatory.

Between the lectures on empathy and the panic over finances, we did have one foray into "Clinical Skills." The university, in its infinite wisdom, decided that before we could be trusted with sharp objects or drugs, we needed to master the art of "Personal Care." Specifically, shaving.

We were herded into the skills suite, a room that smelled faintly of floor polish and desperation. The university had brought in "volunteers." I have no idea who these men were or what dark path in life had led them to volunteer their faces to a room full of petrified students, but there they sat, waiting to be groomed.

There was, however, a logistical issue. The university budget had apparently been blown on the "Empowerment" slides, leaving the cupboard bare of actual clinical supplies. There was no shaving foam. There were no razors. A tutor returned from the canteen, triumphant, clutching a tub of double cream and a box of wooden tongue depressors. "Right," they announced, deadpan. "Improvise." I stared at the tub. We were about to engage in dairy-based personal care. I thought about asking if we should complete an allergies assessment but thought better of it.

I paired up with my friend, a look of pure horror shared between us. We approached our volunteer, a stoic man who looked like he was regretting every life choice he had made since the late seventies. I dipped my gloved hand into the tub. It was thick, rich, and smelled like a scone that had gone wrong. I smeared the double cream onto his chin. He didn't flinch. He closed his eyes, accepting his fate as a human dessert.

Then came the "shave." I picked up the tongue depressor. For the uninitiated, this was a blunt piece of wood usually used to gag children while looking at their tonsils. It had the cutting power of a spoon. I proceeded to scrape the wood through the cream. It didn't shave him; it just redistributed the fat across his jowls. It was like trying to plaster a wall with a lolly stick. The chafe made a sound like sandpaper on leather. "Gentle strokes," the tutor advised, as I effectively exfoliated a stranger using ingredients from a trifle.

Behind us, another pair of students were attempting the "Log Roll" using glide sheets that looked suspiciously like repurposed bay curtains. They were heaving each other back and forth like sacks of potatoes on slippery nylon, trying to maintain dignity while one student's face was gaining friction burns from the vinyl mattress.

I looked at the cream. I looked at the stick. I looked at the volunteer, who was now glazing over like a doughnut. This was higher education. I concluded then that nursing wasn't all about the clinical. It was about maintaining a straight face when the world had gone bat shit crazy. If I could shave a man with a dessert ingredient without cracking a smile, I could probably handle anything.

***

Miraculously, the university administration seemed to have located its own backside with both hands. That "endearing trait" of chaotic disorganisation began to recede, replaced by something resembling competence. We received our next placement allocations before the term ended, which in national health machine time management was equivalent to receiving a letter before you had sent it.

There was less wailing and gnashing of teeth this time around. We had all reached a state of cynical acceptance. We knew how the lottery worked now. You would inevitably be sent somewhere you didn't want to go, to work in a speciality you had zero interest in, located in a town you couldn't find on a map.

We accepted our fate. It was a placement. It was twelve weeks of free labour. It was a learning curve. And as I told myself while staring at the allocation email, even a disaster was educational. Sometimes a placement teaches you how to be a great nurse, and sometimes it teaches you exactly what kind of nurse you never want to become.

My brief flicker of optimism was extinguished the moment I read the location. It was a Community Hospital, a vital local hub that included a Minor Injuries Unit. The list of specialities was exhaustive: skin, gut, liver, joints, eyes. It was backed up by imaging, scanning, and even minor procedure rooms. It was a purpose-built, state-of-the-art facility, the kind of polished healthcare environment that most students only dream of seeing because they were so few and far between. So why did my stomach drop through the floor? Why the sudden dread?

You will find out in the next chapter. But I can tell you now that it had nothing to do with the clinical rotation. The learning opportunity was vast. The hospital purpose built. The problem? It wasn't just a hospital. It was territory.

04

How to Be a Student Nurse and

Be Unapologetically You

Placement two, day one. I walked in with the standard-issue mixture of nausea and blind panic, having absolutely no idea what to expect. As you know already my father was a Charge Nurse for over thirty years. I am not sure whether to say fortunately or unfortunately at this point. The Hospital I had been placed in was his stomping ground for a majority of his career.

To be a black man in a rural provincial backwater during the seventies, eighties and nineties was to be conspicuous. To be a black man in a position of authority, with a white wife and a brood of mixed-race children trailing behind him, was to be a local landmark. We were not your typical family. We were a topic of conversation. We were a walking controversy to be dissected in the smoking area and judged behind closed curtains. Everyone knew us, knew of us, or had a firm opinion on our existence. Now I was walking back into the goldfish bowl.

My introduction, however, caught me completely off guard. I was intercepted at the door by Ms K, a high-ranking deity in the Trust management pantheon. She walked me through the communal areas and the locker room with the brisk efficiency of an estate agent trying to hide damp, before marching me towards the staff room for the morning handover.

Walking into that room felt exactly like stumbling into a remote country pub where the jukebox cuts out the second a stranger enters. The door hinges screamed for oil, announcing my arrival to the room like a fanfare of rusty trumpets. Every head swivelled. Every conversation died. Twenty pairs of eyes locked onto me as if I was carrying a contagious disease or a tax audit.

I tried to sidle towards the back wall, attempting to compress my molecular structure into something invisible. It was a futile effort. Ms K's voice boomed across the silence, bouncing off the linoleum. "Before you all disperse," she announced, beaming. "It is with great pleasure that I introduce our new Student Nurse, Victoria Hinds. I am sure you will all remember her father. He was an integral part of this Hospital for many, many years. He saw us through trials and tribulations and was a core strength for his time here." She gestured to me like a prize heifer at a county show. "We are very proud that you are here to continue your father's legacy, Victoria. We welcome you to the team."

Fuck. Fuck. Fuck. Fuck. Fuck.

No pressure, then. Just thirty years of history and a saint-like reputation to live up to while I tried not to kill anyone with a bed pan.

So, a few weeks into the placement, the initial paralysis began to fade. Supported by a mentor who had the patience of a saint and the oversight of a hawk, I started to find my rhythm. I wasn't just the "daughter of" anymore; I was becoming a functional part of the team, prepping for procedures and navigating the day-to-day chaos without hyperventilating. However, as I got comfortable with the clinical side of things, I started to pay more attention to the social dynamics.

Nurses have opinions. Lots of them. Some are professional and evidence based on things such as wound care or drug interactions. Others are personal. Deeply, viciously personal. There is a strange psychological phenomenon in Hospitals involving bed curtains. We treat these flimsy sheets of fabric as if they are lead-lined walls. We act as though pulling that clinical blue polymer screen around a bed creates a cone of silence, an impermeable fortress where sound goes to die. If the old adage says the walls have ears, then Hospital curtains have unparalleled hearing and a direct line to the gossip column.

It was after the lunch lull and I was in the bed space nearest the hub, quietly prepping a patient for a specialist instillation. The patient was drifting in and out of a chemically induced nap, so I moved with exaggerated stealth, checking the inventory and laying out the equipment on the trolley like a phlebotomist meticulously lining up Vacutainers for a difficult bleed. Because I was silent, I became invisible. The rest of the team were huddled at the hub for the afternoon briefing, and I kept one ear cocked towards them, trying to glean a vague idea of the itinerary I was missing. The clinical handover was informative. The unauthorised addendum that followed was enlightening. My ears pricked up when a hushed voice cut through the scratching of pens. "What do you think of the new student nurse, Vicki, then?"

My spine stiffened. I was immediately annoyed. My name is Victoria. It is not difficult to remember. It is four syllables. I always introduce myself as Victoria. When people take a hatchet to it and shorten it without permission, I usually resort to my standard defence mechanism: I feign total deafness until they correct themselves.

I froze over the sterile pack, realising this wasn't a slip of the tongue. It was a deliberate resize. "I'm not sure about her yet," another voice murmured, dripping with condemnation. "But she obviously thinks she's bloody entitled. I mean, who calls themselves Victoria?" The character assassination didn't end there. It was the warm-up act. "I can't work her out," the voice continued, shrill and confident. "Did you hear her at lunch, banging on about The Boy? She reckons he's about to go to high school. The maths doesn't add up." A pause. A sharp intake of breath. "Either she's got herself The Boy as a stepson, or she got knocked up when she was thirteen."

Group laughter prevailed. It wasn't a warm sound. It was the sound of a clique closing ranks. "Talking of being entitled," another chipped in, "she probably thinks she knows it all just because her Dad worked here a million years ago. Daddy's little princess coming back to the manor." More laughter. Louder this time.

I felt a ball of anxious bile rise from my stomach, burning its way up my oesophagus. It sat in my throat like a swallowed stone. I could feel the capillaries in my cheeks dilating, a hot flush of adrenaline and humiliation creeping up my neck. I stood there, clutching a kidney dish, paralysed by a three-way split decision: laugh out loud, vomit on my shoes, or cry in frustration.

I decided on the first option. The nuclear option. I took a breath deep enough to inhale the entire room, gripped the fabric, and swung the curtains open with the dramatic flair of a magician revealing a tiger. The plastic runners screamed along the track. Swish. The laughter was severed instantly. Four faces turned to me, pale and frozen, like guilty shift workers caught in the clinical glare of an unannounced inspection. I took a moment. I let the silence hang there, heavy and suffocating, soaking in their rising panic.

I offered them a manic, unhinged smile. "Is there anything any of you would like to ask me directly?" The dead air in the room was dense enough to chew. Nobody moved. Nobody breathed. I turned and walked away with purpose, with the muffled squelch of duty shoes on the industrial grade flooring. I decided to count it as a victory. After all, despite the slander, the bitchiness, and the accusation of juvenile delinquency, I walked away pleased with one undeniable fact. They all thought I looked like I was in my mid-twenties.

That was my inaugural baptism into the toxic sludge of the Service "office gossip." What truly winded me wasn't the malice. It was the rank of the participants. This wasn't a gaggle of bored students or a huddle of healthcare assistants blowing off steam. This was a summit meeting of the elite. We are talking Staff Nurses, Sister, and even the visiting Consultant Specialist. The people responsible for life, death, and clinical governance were standing there, tearing a student to shreds within earshot of the day bay. Patients were sitting metres away in paper gowns, waiting for minor ops, listening to the medical team speculate on the timing of my conception.

It was a valuable educational moment, though. I immediately filed three new protocols into my mental handbook: One: When it comes to gossip, assume everyone is capable. The sweet grandmotherly auxiliary and the stone-faced specialist are both susceptible to the dopamine hit of a rumour. Two: Trust no one. Information is ammunition. If you do not want it broadcast on the site Tannoy, do not whisper it in the sluice room. Three: Do not get involved. Stay Switzerland. Neutrality is the only shield you have.

Despite the social minefield, the clinical work was a goldmine. The beauty of a Community Hospital is that it functions like the Swiss Army Knife of the Service. It is geared up for everything: minor injuries, imaging, and specialist-led clinics spanning every discipline from maternity services to end of life care.

I can quite honestly say that this placement was the foundation slab of my entire career. It wasn't all about passing exams; it was a crash course in the gory reality of anatomy, physiology, and the pharmacy's worth of medications required to keep the human body functioning. I learned how to treat the ailment, manage the chronic decay, and navigate the endless paperwork that accompanies both.

It offered a unique vantage point on the patient pathway. In a large teaching centre, you see a trailer. Here, I saw the whole film. I witnessed the entire arc from the initial tentative diagnosis to the final discharge letter. On one occasion, I watched the timeline run from diagnosis to the zipped black bag. I saw the inner workings of the Service stripped bare. I saw its quiet, brilliant successes. And I saw, with uncomfortable clarity, its many, many failures.

Little did I know, I was about to develop a borderline fetish for the shedding of human casing. My next rotation was Dermatology. The unit was run by a coven of specialist nurses who possessed a passion I had previously thought reserved only for religious zealots. They could diagnose a vague patch of red skin in seconds, muttering dead languages like Erythema Multiforme or Keratosis Pilaris as if casting a spell. They wielded an arsenal of magical creams and potions, including tars, steroids, and emollients, which ranged in texture from "luxury moisturiser" to "industrial road lubricant."

If you are the sort of person who derives a sordid thrill from pimple popping, blackhead mining, or the aggressive removal of organic debris, this place was Disneyland. It was a hunting ground for scraping, squeezing, and dry-freezing mysterious skin crustaceans with the violent hiss of liquid nitrogen. Suture removal became a daily ritual. The clinic operated a revolving door for a very specific demographic: elderly men currently paying the invoices for decades of scalp abuse.

A significant portion of our workload consisted of removing stitches from the shiny, mottled domes of men who had spent the last forty years in aggressive denial about their baldness. They seemed to operate under the delusion that three wisps of comb-over provided adequate UV protection. They did not. A hat or a dollop of Factor 50 would have saved them a lot of pain, but in this demographic, sun protection is viewed with deep suspicion.

Around here, being able to "handle the heat" is seen as a masculine endurance sport, ranked alongside drinking 8% beer and eating a vindaloo without sweating. Admitting you need a hat is tantamount to admitting you need a lie-down.

It wasn't only the men, though. The mentality reminded me of the patients who came in with early-stage carcinomas, openly admitting they used baby oil to "accelerate" their tan. They would spend two Weeks a year on a package holiday resort marinating themselves in grease and baking in thirty-eight-degree heat until they resembled rotisserie chickens. Then they would return home to spend the other fifty weeks of the year indoors, fully clothed, wondering why their skin was trying to kill them.

Of course, I had to bite my tongue. I had to keep my expression a solid neutral while I lectured them on sun safety. The irony was thick enough to choke on. In a previous life, before the calling, the poverty, and the uniform, I had been an operator in the engine room of industry. One of my ventures was a tanning shop.

I wasn't a bystander to this carnage. I was the supplier. For years, I had happily taken money from people desperate to turn themselves the colour of a mahogany sideboard. I had sold minutes of UV radiation like sweets in a pick-and-mix. Now, here I was on the other side of the transaction, scrubbing up to surgically remove the consequences of my own former trade. It felt less like nursing and more like serving a very specific, Karmic penance.

Then the time arrived. My turn. My mentor approached me with the grave expression of a priest delivering last rites. "I've made a mistake," she confessed. My brain immediately began cycling through the greatest hits of skin negligence. Oh God, I thought. Have you chemically burned a patient's face? Have you sliced off a healthy earlobe during a biopsy? Have you frozen the wrong pensioner with the liquid nitrogen? But no. It was merely an administrative screw-up. She had double-booked two suture removals for the same slot. "How can I help?" I asked, masking my relief. She replied with the calm, predatory confidence of a veteran who has spent years dumping tasks on juniors. "I need you to do Mr C while I do Mr D in the next cubicle. I'll be right here if you need anything. You've seen a tonne of them, you'll be fine."

Seen a tonne of them? "Seen" was the operative word in that sentence. As for "a tonne," I did a quick mental calculation. A metric tonne is one thousand kilograms. If we assume one observed procedure weighs roughly a kilo, her estimation was out by a factor of about nine hundred and ninety. I hadn't seen a tonne. I had seen a handful. And I had performed exactly zero.

However, I am not one to baulk at a challenge, largely because I am too terrified to say no. I began mentally preparing myself, setting up the sterile field and cracking open the suture removal pack with hands that I prayed weren't shaking.

The ward clerk breezed through, handed us the respective notes, and pointed us towards the waiting area. Mr C. Routine suture removal, post-biopsy, right frontal scalp. Simple enough. I marched out to the waiting room and called his name. "Mr C?" There was no initial answer. Instead, I was intercepted by a woman who seemed to glide rather than walk. She was impeccably dressed and surrounded by a forcefield of stupidly expensive perfume. She didn't smell like the clinic. She smelled of solvency. She smelled of designer scent and condemnation. She possessed an air of grace and decisiveness that made me feel instantly inadequate, a feeling I had experienced before. Specifically, in her presence.

As she moved into the fluorescent light, the penny dropped with the weight of an anvil. It all made sense. Mrs C wasn't just a concerned wife. She was an Honorary Clinical Professor of the university faculty. She was the woman with the authority to sign the paperwork on my degree. I had sat through one of her lectures last term, and now I was about to take a scalpel to her husband's head.

56

Mrs C was a titan of academia. This was a woman whose CV was so extensive it probably required its own ISBN and formal referencing. She exuded pure, unadulterated Headmistress energy. "Ah, a student," she remarked. She gazed at me with an expression that might have been a smile but was statistically more likely to be a grimace.

I immediately engaged my default survival mechanism: aggressive professional deference, otherwise known as brown-nosing. "Mrs C, what a surprise and a pleasure," I lied, extending my hand. She shook it politely, released it, and immediately withdrew a bottle of pocket sanitiser to de-student herself. She scrubbed her palms vigorously, as if my inexperience was a contagious pathogen. "Is it just you?" In the spirit of open, honest transparency, a trait drilled into us at nursing school alongside bed-making and suppressed rage, I replied tentatively.

"Yes, it is. But my mentor is in the cubicle next door for support should it be required."

"Have you seen one?"

"Yes, several."

"Well, it's time for you to do one, then," she stated, effectively sealing the exits. "If it goes well, I'll personally sign off your clinical outcome today. Then you can discuss in the skills lab when you get back to Uni." If it goes well? What did that even mean in this context? What was the worst that could happen? I was removing stitches, not performing open-heart surgery. I wasn't going to accidentally sever an artery. Or was I? Suddenly, a piece of blue nylon thread felt like a loaded weapon.

My progression within Dermatology led me to one of the most inspirational professionals in my career. Ms R was a Nurse Consultant. For those unfamiliar with hierarchy, a Nurse Consultant is a unicorn in a uniform. They are rare, powerful, and usually operate at a level reserved for physicians. She had worked her arse off to become the first Dermatology Nurse Consultant at a major teaching Hospital, paving the road with asphalt so the rest of us could drive on it later.

For reasons that escape me, she took me under her wing. She noticed a spark I didn't recognise in myself. She operated at a surgical level, performing biopsies and micrographic surgery. She didn't just let me watch; she handed me the instruments. On one occasion, she handed me the cryotherapy device, a device for dispensing liquid nitrogen at minus one hundred and ninety-six degrees and let me perform controlled frostbite on a consenting patient. Ms R nurtured not only my knowledge but my fragile confidence. She made me believe this nursing thing could possibly be for me. I still follow her career with awe. She continues to be a battering ram for the profession, proving that nurses can be as clinically lethal as the doctors.

When I thought I had peaked with Ms R, I encountered Mr T. Mr T was a Consultant Surgeon and pain management specialist. Imagine every intimidating stereotype about continental inefficiency distilled into a single human being, and you are halfway there. He had a light, fluid accent and a personality made of velvet. He wore his spectacles high on the bridge of his nose, peering under them with dull brown eyes that demanded absolute silence and attention. He spoke with civilian precision. He did not use unnecessary words. Small talk was a language He refused to learn. If he ever asked you about your weekend, it was likely a diagnostic test for early-onset dementia.

His knowledge was encyclopaedic, but the beautiful thing was that he was a natural teacher. He was infatuated with his specialism and viewed a patient's pain not as a symptom, but as a personal insult he had to defeat. He possessed a yielding, suffocating persistence that made him an angel in a lab coat. Like Ms R, he took me under his wing. I think it was because I asked to follow a patient's treatment pathway from the initial consultation to diagnosis, through to the clinical therapy and the follow-up. Trust me on this one. In this game, enthusiasm is currency. The more questions you ask, the more you learn, and the more doors open. In this case, the door opened to something nothing short of magnificent.

It was a standard Tuesday afternoon of organised chaos. I had apparently proved myself capable enough to be left in charge of running the clinics. This involved herding patients, wrestling medical notes from the filing system, and taking observations for the pre-ops. It was busy, and I was enjoying the responsibility. Then Ms K appeared.

My stomach dropped through the floor. The trepidatious energy returned instantly. Had I killed someone? Had I been rude to a donor? No matter how much experience I gained, I could not shake the Impostor Syndrome rattling my ribcage. I always assumed I was seconds away from being escorted off the premises by security. I braced myself for the dressing down. It didn't come.

"Victoria, I'm taking over from you," Ms K announced. "Mr T has requested your assistance." I stared at him blankly. My brain refused to process the sentence. "Well, go on then," she said, making a shooing motion with her hands like she was displacing a pigeon. "Go and get scrubbed. She is waiting for you in the Day Procedure Unit."

I arrived to find Mr T charming the socks off a patient booked for a carpal tunnel release. There was, however, a significant logistical snag. The patient was a full-time wheelchair user, unable to weight-bear or mobilise. Now, we technically did have hoists, I believed there was one gathering dust somewhere in the depths of Imaging, but before we could organise a search party to retrieve it, the patient intervened.

She had absolutely no interest in being winched out of her chair like a piece of cargo. She cut through the logistical panic with a simple suggestion. She wanted to stay exactly where she was. And, more importantly, she wanted to watch.

Mr T, who never saw a problem he couldn't improvise his way out of, agreed immediately. The patient extended her arm onto the sterile trolley like a queen offering her hand to be kissed. So, there she sat, fully conscious, comfortable in her own chair, peering into the open anatomy of her own wrist while Mr T sliced the transverse carpal ligament. It was macabre, highly irregular, and absolutely staggering.

I was still operating under the assumption that I was purely decorative, there to observe and learn. Mr T had other ideas. He instructed me to get the patient comfortable. Once that was done, he turned to me with a glint in his eye. "Thank you. Now, you have until I have administered the local anaesthetic to scrub in and be ready to assist me."

Assist him?

What the actual fuck?

I froze. My brain had stalled. I turned to the regular scrub team, eyes wide with panic. "What exactly am I supposed to be doing?" The lead scrub nurse looked at me. Her mask was hiding her mouth, but her eyes were crinkling. She was shaking with suppressed mirth. "You're taking lead," she whispered. "You are on retractors."

Retractors?

The metal claws designed to hold the flesh apart. The very instruments that would hold the incision open to provide access to the surgical site. And they were going to be held by me?

60

Panic took the wheel. I scrubbed my hands with a ferocity that nearly took the skin off. The scrub team assisted me into my gown and gloves, which felt positively backwards. It was a violation of the natural order. I was the student, the lowest form of life in the theatre. I should have been gowning them, not the other way around.

To add to the stress, the patient was awake. Fucking awake. There was no dignity screen, no sedative, just a woman actively wanting to watch her own operation in graphic high definition. And that is exactly what happened.

The incision was made. The retractors were in situ, held steady by my own fair hands. Mr T looked up over his spectacles, staring directly into my soul. "Perfect. Now, do not move."

I froze like a statue. Unfortunately, the patient did not. She was so intrigued by the internal mechanics of her own wrist that she decided to take it for a test drive. She started clenching and unclenching her fist, watching the white, pearlescent tendons slide back and forth inside the open wound. It was like watching the arm repair scene in *The Terminator*.

***

Of course, it wasn't all high-fives and open anatomy. I soon learned that patient consent is a volatile variable. I had a brief experience with a patient booked for a Digital Rectal Examination. He took one look at me, a twenty-something female student, and politely but firmly requested I leave the room. He clearly did not want an audience for a DRE. Honestly? I couldn't blame him. It is a vulnerable enough position without having a stranger staring at your undercarriage. I retreated to the corridor without a fuss, accepting that while some patients want to watch their own surgeries, others would quite rightly prefer to keep their dignity intact.

This placement was proving to be far more than a quiet rotation in the sticks. The placement itself was a bit of a phoenix. It had once been a scrappy rural Accident and Emergency Department, a thriving hub of acute care with a long stay ward oddly attached to it. It had metamorphosed into something different. It was now a slick, clinic-led facility supporting specialists diverted from the main teaching Hospital.

The existence of this place was a miracle of inheritance law. It all stemmed from a patient who had received excellent care and, in return, bequeathed a fantastically generous sum of money to the Service. However, this donation came with strings attached. Thick, steel strings. The money had to be spent on that Hospital and only that Hospital.

Naturally, the suits in the ivory towers, likely aided by officials and politicians, hated that. They wanted to sidestep the caveat and dump the cash into the cesspit of the National Health Service budget, where it would inevitably vanish without a trace. The realisation was stark. If that happened, the community would never see a penny of it.

So, a massive legal battle ensued. Everyone knew about it. The local community rallied, armed with petitions and righteous indignation. After public consultation after public consultation, they won. The tired, run-down, not-for-purpose buildings were bulldozed and replaced with the revolutionary care facility I was standing in right then.

It was a triumph of the people over the institution. It just took over a decade to get it done.

Next up was Neuro. By this point, I felt I had chaperoned enough clinics to personally greet half the population of the district, witnessing a dizzying array of medical specialities. However, one particular consultant caught my eye. Simply because she possessed an aura that sucked the air out of the room.

Let's call her Ms P. She was academically published, internationally renowned, and monolithic. The embarrassing part is that, initially, I had absolutely no idea who she was. I treated her like a normal human being. That was a mistake.

I learned my lesson the hard way when I breezed into her room. She sternly informed me that I was to knock, wait for a response, and only then contemplate opening the door. She didn't care if I was holding the coffee she had requested, the patient notes she had screamed for, or news of an impending nuclear strike. Do not enter until summoned. It wasn't a rule. It was law.

I spent hours standing in the corridor like a lemon, clutching a cooling Americano, panicking about the backlog of patients in the waiting room while she finished her consultations at her own glacial pace. It wasn't until I spoke to colleagues that I realised why everyone tiptoed around her. She was one of those people. You know that dinner party question: "Who is the most famous person you've ever met?" In terms of sheer, projected importance? Ms P wins, hands down and I've met Victoria Beckham.

The afternoon clinic was already running on fumes. Ms P had been detained by a medical emergency at the "Mothership", our term for the main teaching Hospital, leaving us with a thirty-minute lag and a waiting room that was rapidly reaching capacity.

I decided to make myself useful. I scrubbed her room down. Aligned the chairs with the precision of a feng shui master. Prepared her coffee exactly as specified, placing it on a coaster to the right of her monitor. I even gambled on a sandwich from the canteen, hoping she didn't have a dairy intolerance.

I retrieved the notes for the first patient, reassured them they hadn't been forgotten, and then stood sentry at the main entrance. I waited. Then I waited some more.

Finally, a sleek black Mercedes AMG came winging it into the car park. Ms P emerged, looking acutely stressed and ready to kill.

She attempted to storm past me.

"Ms P!" I barked.

She spun around, eyes blazing. "WHAT?"

"I have the notes for your first patient. Your room is set up. There is coffee and lunch on your desk." I thrust the medical file into her hand before she could interrupt. "I will be outside your door. Let me know when you are ready to bring the patient through."

She didn't say a word. She snatched the notes and marched inside. Had I saved the day or signed my own death warrant? Fuck knows.

I followed in her slipstream as she marched to her room. She went in and shut the door with a force that rattled the frame. Strictly speaking, site professionals are not supposed to run or slam doors, but apparently those rules did not apply to deities of Neuro.

I took up my post outside. For fear of sounding like a broken record, I waited. I checked my watch. I waited some more. Then, the handle turned. The door opened slowly. The woman who emerged bore no resemblance to the stressed maverick I had met in the car park. She was calm. She was serene. She looked immaculate in a tailored charcoal suit, resembling a Greek goddess who had briefly descended to check on the mortals. She looked at me, seemingly surprised I hadn't fled. "Ah, you really are here," she said softly. "I am ready." I escorted the first patient to the clinic room. I knocked and waited, strictly abiding by the Law, until a bellowed "ENTER" granted us permission.

With the patient safely inside and the immediate crisis averted, I retreated to the hub. I collapsed into a chair and took several deep breaths to lower my heart rate. I knew her appointments usually ran to a strict fifteen minutes. I quickly pulled myself together and retrieved the notes for the second patient. I took up my position and waited dutifully until the first patient emerged. Then, I made my move. Before she could close the door, which would have forced me to endure the knocking ritual for the millionth time, I slipped into the room. I walked in, placed the new file on her desk, and left without saying a single word, closing the door softly behind me. Between patients, clinicians must update their notes both manually and electronically. They must do this in real time. Because they work on a ridiculously pressured time scale, they require a vacuum of silence for optimum concentration.

So, I waited. When the door opened, she looked ready to march out and fetch the patient herself. Instead, she found me standing there like a loyal guard dog. "Oh, you're here?" more than surprised. "Yes," I replied. "For the next thirty minutes. Then I have been allocated to Imaging. But I will escort your next patient through now." She didn't say anything. However, by the time that fifteen-minute consultation had concluded, she had already paged Ms K. She had requested me for her entire service for the afternoon. Imaging would have to wait.

All was going surprisingly well. Ms P even attempted a form of stilted conversation. As she was frantically scribbling her notes, she asked, almost absent-mindedly, "So, do you have an interest in Neuro?" "Yes, very much," I replied. I was careful to keep it brief. I suffer from skittish, verbal diarrhoea, and once the dam breaks, I cannot stop. I suspected Ms P was not a fan of chatter. "Hmm," she murmured. "If you get consent from my remaining patients, you can sit in for their consultations." Bloody hell!

I simply said, "Thank you," and walked out with the dignity of a saint. Inwardly, however, I was screaming. I was doing the imaginary Carlton dance from *The Fresh Prince of Bel-Air* down the entire length of the corridor. But then, trouble struck on the second patient. Why was it always me?

Ms P was a vertical presence at six feet and taller than me which is a rarity. She stood towering over both the patient and his wife, a petite woman barely five feet tall who was clutching her husband's arm with a grip that was turning his skin white. They were trembling with anxiety, awaiting the verdict. Ms P flicked through the notes. "I can confirm that you have Parkinson's Disease." She didn't even look up from the pages. The patient was mute. He was forty-seven. He had a long life ahead of him, and the rug had been pulled out. His wife remained silent, but heavy, bulbous tears began to roll down her cheeks, splashing onto her lap and the floor.

Ms P, oblivious to the emotional bomb she had detonated, turned to her computer. She began tapping the keys wildly, listing medications that required a PhD to pronounce and suggesting lifestyle adjustments as if she were reading a shopping list. The couple were distraught, not given a single second to process the devastation. It was heart-wrenching. I had to do something. I stood up from my corner, walked to the desk, and committed a cardinal sin. I reached right across Ms P, violating her sacred personal space, to grab the box of tissues. I handed them to the wife.

Ms P stopped typing. She looked at me as if I had slapped her. But then, her gaze followed the tissues. She looked at the patient. She looked at the weeping wife. She paused. She sat back in her chair. The glare softened into something resembling an epiphany. "Ah," she said.

"Would you both like a minute?" They nodded profusely. Ms P turned to me. "Take them to the canteen for a coffee. Escort them back in twenty minutes while I prepare some literature."

I dutifully did so, terrified of the retribution that awaited me for my silent, but very public, insubordination. We returned to find a transformed Ms P. She was less Consultant, more human. She walked them through their options with patience, gave them time to think, and provided the contact details for her Advanced Practice Nurse for ongoing support. The tears had dried, and while the couple were undoubtedly still stunned, they were no longer distraught. They thanked her and left.

Ms P called me back in. My stomach turned over. I braced myself for the inevitable bollocking. I expected a lecture on "overstepping the mark" or a reminder of my lowly status in the food chain. Instead, she looked at me wearily. "Thank you for that, Victoria. Sometimes I get so consumed with the clinical that I overlook the patient." She then shooed me out of the room, returning to her notes as if the moment of vulnerability had never happened. I left without a word, buzzing. Not only was I not in trouble, but the Goddess of Neuro had remembered my name.

Bagging a position in a hospital like this is the nursing equivalent of arriving at a hotel and being upgraded to the Presidential Suite just because you had the audacity to ask. We are talking about the full package. King-sized bed, sea view, and a complimentary mini bar.

Compared to the crumbling Victorian workhouses I was used to, this place was a sanctuary. It offered beautiful modern architecture, state-of-the-art equipment, and staff facilities that rivalled a high-end spa. But the real luxury? The hours. We were open from 08:00 to 17:00. Let that sink in. It meant the same standard salary, but with zero twelve-hour shifts, barely any personal care, and absolutely no back-breaking manual handling. All within normal business hours. No nights. No weekends. No Bank Holidays.

Safe to say, if you want to land a job in a utopia like this, you need to start preparing now. Work your arse off, secure a top-tier degree, and build a CPD portfolio that would put Daphne Steel to shame.

As I packed up my things, there were the usual pleasantries. "Don't be a stranger" and "Don't forget us when you qualify, there will always be a job here for you."

So, that was a wrap. Community Hospital Placement done. Did I continue my father's legacy? I doubt it. But I like to think I carved out a little piece of my own.

05

How to Be a Student Nurse and

Wear Two Uniforms

The academic calendar suggests that life can be organised into neat, manageable blocks. Term one. Winter break. Term two. It implies a rhythm, a structure where you learn, you rest, and you return refreshed with a new set of stationery and an optimistically clean notebook. My life, however, preferred the "clusterfuck" approach to scheduling. As I had scraped together enough serotonin to simulate a positive attitude for the new term, the universe decided I looked a bit too relaxed and lobbed a grenade at my head.

I wasn't sure if fate was timing these disasters to ensure I was match-fit enough to handle them, or if I was simply too anaesthetised by the sheer exhaustion of placement to notice the walls caving in until the rubble physically hit me. This particular catastrophe arrived in the form of a formal interview.

The event in question had occurred right before my induction at the university, a dark prologue to my new career that I had tried to edit out of the final cut. The circumstances didn't just haunt me. They sat on my chest at 3am. It was a specific, heavy brand of guilt that I carried around like a backpack filled with lead shot. The Boy had witnessed the incident. He had seen the violence that finally snapped the spine of my previous relationship.

I would never, ever be able to scrub the sound of his voice from my auditory cortex. He screamed "Mummy" at a pitch that bypassed the ear and went straight to the bone marrow. He was petrified. He was a child. And yet, amidst the chaos, he was the one who had the presence of mind to dial the emergency number.

I had always cultivated a self-image of resilience. I liked to think that if cornered, my fight-or-flight mechanism would kick in and I'd go down swinging. I was wrong. In that scenario, physics won. I was overpowered, pinned, and nullified in my own defence. It was possible that The Boy saved my life that night. Not only in the literal sense, because his scream startled the aggressor enough to stop them crushing the air out of my lungs, but in the existential sense too.

That moment was the catalyst. It wasn't a gentle discovery. It was a violent shove. The severity of what he saw gave me the impetus to finally exit a volatile situation I had been blind to for far too long. I couldn't stay for me, but I certainly couldn't stay for him.

The morning after the night that broke everything, the doorbell rang. It was a safeguarding officer. While my then-partner was enjoying the dubious hospitality of the holding cells, I was sitting on my sofa, clutching a mug of tea that I had no intention of drinking, trying to navigate a conversation I never thought I'd need to have. The officers were kind. They were empathetic, supportive, and armed with leaflets. They were firmly of the opinion that abuse, regardless of the postcode or the apologies offered, required a paper trail.

I, conversely, was firmly of the opinion that we should pretend this never happened so I could get on with my life. I was stuck in the "can't we scrub the whiteboard and start over" mindset. Denial is a powerful anaesthetic, but it wears off quickly when someone pulls out a camera.

Having photographs taken of my injuries was a particularly low point. It felt less like an interview and more like a clinical audit of my body. Turn left. Chin up. Hold still. By the time I had stammered out a brief statement, the adrenaline had drained away, leaving the raw, throbbing reality of the situation. The officer, sensing that I was about to dissolve into the onset throws of a mental breakdown right there on the carpet, wisely concluded the interview. They snapped their notebook shut and planned arrangements for a follow-up, treating my emotional collapse with the same efficient triage one might apply to a minor bleed.

My then-partner was still detained. The terms were made explicitly clear: they were not to contact me, they were not to come within a certain radius of my front door, and if they wanted their pants and toothbrush, they would need an escort to retrieve them.

Everything went quiet after that. In the weeks that followed, the silence from their end was absolute, so I did what any sane, traumatised student nurse would do. I took the entire incident, wrapped it in mental hazard tape, and shoved it to the very back of my mind. I knew, logically, that I needed to process it. I knew I needed to grieve, to heal, to sit in a circle and talk about my feelings. But I had anatomy exams to pass and The Boy to raise. I simply didn't have the diary space for a breakdown. Was it a healthy psychological strategy? Absolutely not. Was it necessary for survival? Without a doubt.

The correspondence arrived sporadically, landing on my doormat like unexploded ordnance. I developed a specific aversion to brown envelopes with official crests. Some I engaged with, offering the bare minimum of cooperation required to keep them at bay, while others I ignored in their entirety. I slid them into a drawer unopened as if they were final demands for a TV licence I didn't have. I wanted it finished. I wanted the credits to roll so I could leave the cinema.

I was trapped in a paradox of my own making. On one hand, I was furious at the prospect of them getting away with it, of walking free to ruin someone else's life. On the other hand, the thought of subjecting myself, and more importantly The Boy, to the callous brutality of the court system was nauseating. So I continued to employ the "Ostrich Strategy." I unrealistically pretended that if I kept my head buried in the sand long enough, the problem would dissipate on its own accord.

I was blind to the severity of the situation because I chose to be. My brain started churning out excuses in a desperate attempt to protect itself. I found myself performing mental gymnastics to create feasible explanations to alleviate the guilt. Then, the decision was taken out of my hands.

I received a notification that the prosecution service was proceeding with the case. They didn't need my permission. They didn't need my statement. They were prosecuting with or without my direct support. The news hit me with a complex cocktail of emotions. There was a heavy dread because I knew this meant the nightmare wasn't over. It was going to be dragged out through hearings and legal arguments. Yet, underneath the dread, there was a profound sense of relief. I didn't have to pull the trigger. The gun had been taken away from me, and the law enforcers were firing it on my behalf.

The silence, as it turned out, was merely a ceasefire. Shortly after the notification, the floodgates didn't just open. They were blown off their hinges. My ex, in a state of desperation, decided that the risk of breaching their conditions was far outweighed by the permanent stain of a criminal record for assault occasioning actual bodily harm. They did the maths and decided harassing me was worth the gamble.

The messages started as a trickle. They crept into my phone with feigned apologies. You know the genre. The "I'm sorry you feel that way" texts. The ones that said all the right words in the correct order but were totally devoid of accountability or remorse. I ignored them. I let the phone buzz and vibrate like an angry wasp, refusing to pick it up. I simply didn't have the bandwidth to deal with it.

When the soft approach failed, they pivoted to the "do you know what this will do to me" strategy. This was their trump card. With a criminal record of this nature, they would inevitably lose their job. The specifics of their employment required a clean sheet, and a domestic abuse conviction was a career-ending event. They hammered this point home relentlessly. They banged on about being homeless, jobless, and destitute, claiming they had no money for legal representation.

They had mastered the art of manipulation to a level that was almost impressive. They could twist reality like a balloon animal until it looked like something decidedly different. Every message was spun to imply that I was the architect of their downfall. If I hadn't reported it, they wouldn't be in this mess. They should have been a politician. They had that unique ability to speak absolute fiction with the conviction of absolute truth.

The gaslighting began to seep in. Was I angry with him that night? Yes. Did I argue with him? Yes. But did I deserve a beating? Definitely not. My logical brain knew this. My emotional brain, however, was battered and easily confused. I had to keep manifesting a mantra to persuade myself, repeating it over and over as I stared at the ceiling in the dark. It was not my fault.

The phone wasn't just buzzing anymore; it was radiating radioactive levels of toxicity. The messages shifted gears from pathetic pleas to aggressive accusations. They were firing off conjecture and threats with the manic energy of a person who knows the walls are closing in. The tension was tangible. It sat in my jaw, grinding my molars down to stumps. I had run out of tears days ago. My tear ducts were dusty, leaving only a cold, functional rage.

I called my liaison officer. I didn't ask for advice. I demanded an intervention. They were efficient. They contacted my ex immediately to reiterate the terms of their conditions in words of one syllable. Cease all contact or risk further arrest.

The direct messages stopped abruptly. But narcissists are like mould. If you bleach one corner, they bloom somewhere else. He couldn't get to me directly, so he started a proxy war. I noticed a digital culling. The numbers on my social media friends lists started dropping. Mutual acquaintances, people I had cooked for and laughed with, began blocking me. I was clearly the villain of the week at his local pub. I could picture him holding court at the bar, spinning a tale of victimhood to anyone who would buy him a pint.

Then came the public posts. The "vague booking." He started sharing those profound quotes that usually accompany a picture of a sunset or a lion. One particularly nauseating example read, "My side of the story doesn't matter anymore. Life happened, it hurt, I healed, but most importantly I learned who deserves a seat at my table and who will never sit at it again."

It was the kind of self-aggrandising drivel that usually signals a guilty conscience. It was a desperate attempt to garner sympathy from the cheap seats. Honestly, I didn't give two shits. If those people wanted a seat at his table, they were welcome to the indigestion. As far as I was concerned, the trash was taking itself out.

A few days passed in relative silence. I was lured into a false sense of security, foolishly believing that the soul-destroying messages were over. I thought the infection had been treated and the antibiotics were working. That delusion lasted a hot minute.

Then came the onslaught.

It wasn't him this time. It was the cavalry. I knew he was persuasive, but holy shit, this was another level of radicalisation. He had mobilised his entire gene pool. His parents got involved. His siblings got involved. Even his in-laws, people who technically had no skin in the game, decided to weigh in on my moral character. The only members of his clan who didn't join the crusade were his own children.

He had somehow, miraculously, managed to raise them into grown-arse adults with more sensibility than he possessed in his little finger. This was likely because he had been estranged from them for years after treating their mother with the same disdain he had eventually shown me. I should have seen that as a massive, neon-lit red flag. Instead, I had viewed it as a "complicated past." Hindsight is a wonderful diagnostic tool, isn't it?

The messages from his family followed a predictable script. They started with the guilt trips. "What are you doing this for?" and "You're going to ruin him," as if I had dragged him out of his house and forced him to destroy his own life. But as I failed to engage, the tone darkened. The pleas turned into sinister warnings. "Karma is a bitch," one auntie texted, followed by vague assertions that "terrible things" were going to happen to me.

It was the final message, a concise and charming "Fuck off and die," that forced my hand. That wasn't harassment. That was a threat.

I went back to the police. I added another layer to the file. And then, I instituted a scorched-earth policy. I didn't just ignore them; I surgically removed them. I deleted and blocked anyone and everyone I had ever come into contact with via him. If they had his surname or had ever been tagged in a photo with him, they were gone. It was a digital amputation, and it was the only way to stop the gangrene from spreading.

Although my personal life was currently resembling a smoking crater, I still managed to drag my husk to university every morning. My logic was simple. I might be functioning on 10% battery power and crying in the toilets during break, but I would have 100% attendance. I couldn't control the court case, but I could control the register. It was one less stick for the university to beat me with.

That term, the curriculum pivoted to shared practice (interprofessional learning). Usually, this is the sort of corporate team-building exercise that makes you want to gnaw your own arm off to escape, but it was the first learning experience I really felt enthused about. It involved herding a gaggle of wannabe healthcare professionals from a myriad of faculties, including medical students, physio students, social workers, and nurses, into one room and forcing us to play nice. We were tasked with formulating a healthcare plan for a real-life case study, simulating a multi-agency team meeting.

The concept was sound. The execution, however, came with a caveat that struck fear into the heart of every British introvert.

Role play.

We were asked to 'play the role' and discuss the case as if we were already qualified professionals who had built a therapeutic relationship with the patient. It required a suspension of disbelief that I wasn't sure I possessed, but I strapped on my imaginary epaulettes and got on with it.

Our patient was 'D'. The brief described him as a 69-year-old male who had been living with insomnia for the past eight years, managed, or rather mismanaged, with Temazepam. The clinical picture was messy. Symptoms included sweating, agitation, confusion, tremors, light sensitivity, and pacing. The backstory was as grim; loss of employment had left him feeling defunct, stripped of his identity. Crucially, although the prescription had recently ceased, D had been supplementing and self-administering his medication. Aware of the spiralling issue and prompted by a worried spouse, assistance had finally been sought via a primary care appointment.

The cast was assembled. We had a GP, me playing the Community Nurse, a Mental Health Nurse, and a Social Worker. An administrative coordinator sat poised with a pen, acting as the scribe.

We sat around a circular table, a geometry doubtless chosen to imply non-hierarchical equality. We went around the circle, introducing ourselves by name and fictitious title. It felt ridiculous, like bad amateur dramatics, but we had to commit to the bit.

Having already completed two sessions, the initial awkwardness had faded. This wasn't a tick-box exercise anymore. When we opened the file on D, the mood in the room shifted. This was a 69-year-old man whose life had unravelled, the loose thread being an eight-year prescription that had spiralled out of control. The scenario felt heavy. It felt real.

The student playing the GP cleared their throat. They had clearly practised this. Their voice was calm, methodical, and pitched about an octave lower than usual to convey authority.

"Thank you all for joining at short notice," they began, smoothing out their notes. "We're here to discuss patient D. As you know from my referral, he is a 69-year-old male who presented recently with his spouse as support."

They paused for effect, scanning the room to ensure we were all paying attention.

"He's been prescribed Temazepam to treat the signs and symptoms relating to insomnia for the better part of eight years. Recently, following a job loss, he began supplementing his dose. Then, prompted by concern from his spouse, he ceased it abruptly." They looked up, grave and serious. "The man I saw was in significant distress caused by acute benzodiazepine withdrawal."

I scribbled 'eight years' on my notepad and underlined it twice. That wasn't a prescription; that was a dependency. Going cold turkey on an eight-year benzo habit wasn't just "distress." It was a physiological derailment.

The GP pressed on, outlining the classic, severe presentation of withdrawal.

"Sweating, visible tremors, agitation, and profound confusion," they listed, counting them off on their fingers. "His spouse mentioned he's been pacing relentlessly and is now highly sensitive to light."

It sounded less like a medical history and more like an exorcism. The body was screaming for the chemical hook it had clung on to for eight years.

"The core psychological stressor appears to be becoming unemployed," they added, glancing at the Social Worker. "Which has left him feeling, in his own words, 'completely useless'."

That part stuck. Take away a man's purpose, remove the structure of his day, and then strip away the medication that numbs the silence? It was a recipe for disaster. It wasn't only a loss of income; it was an amputation of utility.

The GP summarised their clinical rationale with impressive confidence. "I've stabilised him by commencing an equivalent dose of Diazepam. It's a long-acting agent that will give us a much smoother foundation for a very slow, structured taper."
They paused, letting the pharmacology sink in. Temazepam leaves the system quickly, creating peaks and troughs that wreak havoc on the brain. Diazepam is the gentle slope. It was the textbook play.

"My immediate concern was preventing a seizure," they continued, dropping the reality that usually makes students sit up straighter. Benzo withdrawal is more than uncomfortable; it can be fatal. "Now, we need a robust, wraparound plan."

Ah, the "wraparound plan." That was a full house on my NHS Buzzword Bingo card.

They turned their gaze to me. "Community Nurse, you made the initial home visit yesterday. What was your assessment?"

It was my cue. I looked down at my notes. Having not done that placement yet, I was flying blind, channelling a mix of hospital discharge summaries and common sense to fill the role.

"I saw D at home yesterday afternoon," I began, hoping I sounded authoritative. "The physical symptoms track exactly with what the GP has described. He is tachycardic with a resting heart rate sitting at 108 bpm. The tremor is pronounced; it's significant enough that he can't hold a cup of tea without scolding himself somewhere."

I pictured the scene I was inventing. The gloom. The smell of stale air.

"The environment is effectively locked down," I continued. "The curtains were drawn tight in every room due to his photophobia. It felt more like a bunker than a bungalow. His spouse is doing their best, but they're visibly fraying at the edges. They admitted they feel out of their depth. They're more than a spouse right now; they're an untrained mental health nurse, and they're terrified." I paused. I needed them to see the man, not the addict.

"The agitation was extreme," I said. "He couldn't sit still. He paced the living room the entire time, telling me he felt like a caged animal and his brain wouldn't switch off."

79

I glanced at the others. "The shame was palpable. He feels he's failed his spouse."

I checked my list, keeping the plan concise. "My immediate strategy is twice-weekly visits to monitor observations and progress using CIWA-B. They need psychoeducation, they need to know this is chemical, not moral, and a single point of contact so they don't feel abandoned."

The student playing the Mental Health Nurse was next. They flipped through their notebook, adopting an expression of pensive concern.

"Thank you, Nurse," they said. "That paints a very clear picture. We're seeing two issues running in parallel here; the physiological withdrawal and a profound psychological dependency."

They looked up, delivering their analysis with conviction. "For eight years, Temazepam hasn't just been to aid sleep. It's been his primary tool for managing anxiety. Now that tool is gone, and he's been plunged into a personal crisis with the loss of his professional identity. The insomnia he is experiencing is the symptom, not the disease."

The Mental Health Nurse continued, clearly warming to their theme.

"My priority is to build a therapeutic alliance," they stated, hitting the buzzword with a firm emphasis. "He needs a safe space to process these feelings of uselessness without judgement. Initially, our sessions will focus strictly on stabilisation and grounding techniques. These are simple tools he and his spouse can use when the anxiety peaks."

They tapped their pen on the table. "Once the acute withdrawal settles, we can introduce a structured course of Cognitive Behavioural Therapy for Insomnia. The goal is to give him the skills to manage sleep and anxiety for good, but we can't overwhelm him with the heavy lifting right now. He needs a life raft before he can learn to swim."

Listening to the Mental Health Nurse, the logic of the multidisciplinary approach started to make sense. I could see how my visits would act as the scaffolding for their work. While they taught the theory, I could reinforce the practice. I could remind D of the grounding techniques while I was taking his blood pressure, bridging the gap between the sanitised safety of a therapy session and the messy reality of trying to cope in his own living room.

The Social Worker spoke next. Their focus shifted away from the biochemistry and towards the world outside D's curtains.

"That word 'useless' from the primary care consultation is the key for me," they said, leaning forward to emphasise their point. "This isn't just a medical or psychological issue. It is an existential one. D has lost his routine, his social network, and his sense of purpose. A prescription can't fix that."

They continued, outlining a strategy that was refreshingly practical.

"I'll make contact this week to conduct a full social assessment." "We need to ensure he's receiving every penny of financial support he's entitled to. Money worries are a massive stressor, and alleviating that pressure is a quick win." They glanced down at the patient profile. "More importantly, I want to excavate his skills. He was a skilled tradesperson, I believe? There are local groups, such as a men's workshop network, that are brilliant for channelling practical skills and fostering peer support. It gets men out of the house and into a workshop. It is not about replacing his job. It is about helping him construct a new identity that has value."

We all nodded in unison. It was the collective agreement of a team that had successfully navigated a hypothetical crisis without the patient being sectioned.

The GP moved to wrap things up. "Excellent," they said. "This is exactly the kind of multi-pronged approach he needs. So, the plan is set. I will manage the Diazepam taper, but Community Nurse and I will be relying on your feedback to guide the pace. If the withdrawal symptoms spike, let us know immediately, and we will hold the dose."

I vocalised my agreement and scribbled the instruction into my notes to add to D's care plan. Patient D was in safe hands.

They looked at each of us in turn, cementing the chain of command with the confidence of someone born to lead a morning briefing.

"Community Nurse, you remain our eyes and ears on the ground." "We need that vital monitoring to ensure safety. Mental Health Nurse, you address the underlying psychological drivers." "And Social Worker, you focus on the rebuild. We need to reconstruct his sense of self-worth and social connection."

They closed the file with a definitive snap. "Let's schedule a review for a couple of weeks. Good work, everyone."

As the meeting concluded and we broke character, the artificiality of the situation fell away. I felt a genuine sense of coordinated purpose. We weren't just throwing pills at a list of symptoms. We were constructing a scaffold. It was a holistic safety net, woven from medical, psychological, and social support, designed to drag the fictional D through the chemical storm of withdrawal and deposit him back on the shores of a meaningful life.

This process did something unexpected to my serotonin levels. I felt professionally recognised. Valued, even. In a life currently defined by chaos and legal threats, this was a rare moment of clarity. I had fathomed, with a jolt of surprise, that despite the madness, I might have found my place in nursing.

Buoyed by this newfound academic confidence, university became the one quadrant of my life that wasn't actively on fire. I clung to that stability. I used the momentum of the term to throw myself back into full-time work hours, fitting shifts around lectures in a desperate attempt to outrun financial suicide.

I kept myself moving. If I stopped, I had to think, and if I thought, I would crumble. I discovered that I could cope with almost anything if I was in a permanent state of exhaustion. Fatigue became my anaesthetic.

However, there was one emotion that no amount of double shifts or academic success could squash.

Loneliness.

It is a specific kind of torture. Every relationship, no matter how toxic it becomes, has good parts. If it didn't, you never would have signed up for it in the first place. Annoyingly, my brain had decided to engage in a cruel act of historical revisionism. It was playing a highlight reel of the "good days" on a loop, conveniently editing out the shouting, the fear, and the authorities.

I loathed doing the simple things I once used to relax. In the past, we had loved cooking together, usually with some music playing and a bottle of red wine breathing on the counter. Now, the kitchen felt like a tomb. With The Boy increasingly absent, working evening shifts in a café and eating his meals there, I couldn't fathom the energy to cook for myself. The joy of food had evaporated. I resorted to sad microwave meals, unhealthy snacks, or often, not eating at all.

We lived a short walk from the sea, and we used to walk along the path in the evenings, dissecting our days and planning a future that no longer existed. Now, without a sounding board or company, the walk felt like a trudge against the wind. Even watching TV became a painful exercise. Belly laughing at a joke, only to turn and realise there was no one there to share it with, made the comedy instantly tragic.

I was slowly becoming a recluse. I found the thought of recreational activity unfulfilling and futile. Despite the court case, despite the terror, I still missed him.

I stopped myself.

Did I?

I interrogated that feeling. I didn't miss the person who had tormented me. I didn't miss the walking on eggshells. The truth settled, with a heavy heart, that I didn't miss him. I missed somebody. I missed the shape of another human being in the room. There is a lot to be said for the company of others; its absence is a noise all of its own.

It was a cruel paradox. I was starving for human connection, yet the very thought of a social situation triggered a rising tide of panic. I was safe within the structured confines of university or the workplace. In those environments, I had a role to play. I had a script. I was 'The Student' or 'The care assistant'. I didn't have to be 'The Woman Whose Life is Falling Apart'.

Consequently, the only people I saw were fellow students or colleagues. I hid in plain sight.

But you cannot hide from student nurses. We are trained to observe, to look for the subtle signs of deterioration, and my core group of friends at university were no exception. They began to notice the cracks in my armour. They saw past the deflection and the manic work ethic. They gently encouraged me to talk, trying to pry open the lid I was keeping so tightly shut. They made a real, concerted effort to break down my walls, constantly trying to invite me out or include me in their plans.

It is the oldest cliché in the self-help book, but it turns out to be infuriatingly true. It wasn't until I finally stopped looking, until I ceased scanning the horizon for a rescuer and decided to save myself, that the shift happened.

I started taking care of me. I began to rebuild the foundations of my self-worth, brick by brick. I learned to not tolerate the silence in the evenings, but to actively attempt to enjoy it. I reached a state of equilibrium where I was utterly uninterested in a relationship. I was closed for business. No vacancies.

And naturally, talk about timing. That is precisely when the universe decided to intervene.

That was when I met him. My best friend who I didn't know at the time was my soul mate. The timing was laughable, almost cosmic in its irony. Just as I decided I was enough on my own, I met the person who would show me what a partnership was supposed to look like. But I am getting ahead of myself. I will introduce you to him in the next book: *Newly Qualified Edition*. He deserves an introduction worthy of the monumental impact he had.

06

How to Be a Student Nurse and

Survive the Sensory Assault

As the academic calendar shed its pages, the stabilisers come off. The placements stopped being "gentle introductions to care" and started feeling more like combat training. The ultimate prize, the endorphin-soaked Holy Grail for the compulsive, was A&E. It was the stomping ground you needed to survive if you wanted to learn the dark arts of the trade. It was the place where you learned to function in a pressure cooker fuelled by acute stress and systemic crisis.

The university, generally, was reluctant to send us there. It was a liability. Sending a bright-eyed fresher to A&E was like sending a toddler to defuse a bomb. The result was usually a catastrophic emotional mess and a sudden transfer to a Philosophy degree before they had even smelled graduation.

But there was a rare, fanatic breed of student that knew from day one they were built for the pit. They were the A&E purists. These mythical beasts were prepared to harass anyone of clout. Ward Managers, Matrons, Chiefs of Staff: even the poor administrative souls in the placement office were fair game. They possessed the persistence of a resistant strain of hospital-acquired infection. They displayed their eagerness like a plumage, desperate to be thrown into the furnace. It was like watching baby "Nurseicorns" hunting for a golden stethoscope whilst completely unaware that the only thing golden in A&E was the septic shower you got when a catheter bag burst.

The faculty insisted that placements were 'potluck'. They claimed it was a randomised lottery designed to ensure fairness across the cohort. This was, of course, an administrative lie. There appeared to be a direct correlation between your academic performance and the severity of the trauma they decided to inflict upon you. I had flagged myself as a liability by being competent. With a high distinction followed by a strong pass across the first two modules, I had inadvertently volunteered for the front line. My reward for this academic excellence was a placement on the Medical Assessment Unit.

If A&E was the fiery impact zone, MAU was the triage tent immediately next to the crater. Every soul walking, limping, or being wheeled through the sliding doors of A&E were sorted into five categories. It was a grim hierarchy of need. You had the 'Immediate' cases, the ones actively trying to shuffle off this mortal coil requiring full-blown resuscitation. Then came the "Very Urgent" and "Urgent" cases, serious conditions that needed rapid intervention before they slid into the first category. Then you had the "Semi-urgent," and finally, the "non-urgent." These were the brutalised "floor sitters." They were the walking wounded, or often the walking worried, whose conditions were not true emergencies and who were eventually filtered out to minor injuries or back to where they came from.

National targets insisted this entire sorting process must be completed within a fixed window. You had read the newspapers. You knew this target was treated with the same reverence as a drunken New Year's resolution. It was a statistical fantasy. Fundamentally, the rule was simple. If the patient didn't need immediate surgery and wasn't quite dead yet, they got shoved sideways to MAU to stop the clock ticking. That was where I would be waiting.

My mentor was a formidable anomaly. She was seasoned, but she possessed a fire in her belly that suggested she ran on jet fuel rather than caffeine. She was efficient, methodical, and held the unnerving ability to remain serenely calm while the world burned around her. She had recently been promoted to a senior band, which in nursing terms meant she was the one holding the keys to all of the drugs cupboards and the responsibility for the chaos. I was not sure there was a single thing she didn't know, from the intricacies of obscure pathophysiology to the dark art of coordinating bed flow.

She was so full of boundless, irritating energy that she spent her days off mucking out kennels and walking dogs. In contrast, I was already spending my days off lying in a cold, dark room, contemplating my own mortality and trying to decompress from the neurological static of the last shift.

On AMU, there was no gentle easing in. The teaching philosophy was the age-old medical mantra: "See one, do one, teach one." It was a concept that sounded efficient in a textbook but was soul-crushing in practice. You watched a procedure once. Then you were handed the sharp object and told to have a go. "Thrown in at the deep end" was a polite understatement. I had been plucked from a chilled-out placements of gentle rehabilitation, therapy pools, and focused breathing, and dropped into the trenches. AMU was a cattle shed full of critically ill human beings. There was no time for holistic care or holding hands. It was a production line of IV access, stat fluids, and the titration of medications so complex that a decimal point error could kill an elephant.

My only theoretical safety net was the rulebook. Technically, as a student nurse, I was not allowed to be unleashed upon the public unsupervised. I was required to be tethered to my allocated mentor, or failing that, another registered nurse with more than a year's experience who was working towards their practice-educator qualification. That was the official line.

In reality, the staffing rota on AMU was usually a skip fire, and the rules were the first thing to burn. You were frequently passed around like a malaise. You would be fobbed off onto the nearest nurse standing still long enough to be tagged, irrespective of their experience, their ability to teach, or their tolerance for wide-eyed novices.

It was hard to blame them for the heavy sigh that usually accompanied my arrival. There were many reasons why nurses avoided students, but the primary one was simple economics: they didn't get paid for it. While some providers made vague promises about career development, in my experience, mentors received exactly zero pounds and zero pence for the privilege of dragging a student through a twelve-hour shift. It slowed them down. It risked their registration. Consequently, people only took students for one of two reasons. Either they were doing it out of the sheer, saintly goodness of their hearts, or they were cynically ticking a box to boost their CV for a senior band promotion.

The Provider I was placed in operated in a very specific, very rural corner of the world. It was known locally as "Retirement Belt," though on bad days we referred to it as "The Departure Lounge." It was a sprawling, logistical nightmare that officially spanned four counties, though depending on which bureaucrat you asked, it bled into a further three. We were talking about 6,942 square miles of winding back roads and isolated care services.

Within this massive geographical footprint, there were ten major hospitals. Nine of them were open to the chaotic intake of A&E. On paper, this sounded robust. In reality, these hospitals offered a combined total of 3,912 beds to serve a population of approximately 1,742,000 people.

You didn't need a degree in statistics to see the chilling discrepancy in those numbers. It was a game of musical chairs where the music never stopped, and the contestants were all octogenarians with fractured necks of femurs. A hospital bed in this Provider was not only valuable; it was ethereal. To describe them as "gold dust" was a cliché that didn't quite capture the desperation. Finding a free bed was like finding a

Golden Ticket to the Chocolate Factory, except the factory was full of hospital-acquired infection and the chocolate was usually a bowel movement.

There was a non-negotiable expectation ingrained in the student contract: They owned your soul, and you would present it for inspection whenever the schedule demanded. We were expected to honour all shifts allocated to us, regardless of whether they clashed with birthdays, weddings, or the primal need for sleep. I had lucked out in my previous placements, somehow managing to swerve the dreaded 'Night Shifts.'

For many students, the night shift was the bogeyman of the degree. They avoided it with a desperation that suggested a genuine fear of a zombie apocalypse, or perhaps a phobia of the specific brand of ghosts that haunted public-health corridors at Stupid O' Clock. To escape the schedule, I had witnessed levels of creativity that would shame a Booker Prize winner. I had seen students claim they needed to provide overnight care for elderly grandparents who, upon closer inspection, died during a past government. I had heard tales of 'selective narcolepsy' that miraculously only presented between the hours of 20:00 and 09:00. I had even heard students claim they could not access public transport at night, despite living in campus accommodation that was literally a stone's throw from the hospital entrance. They could roll out of bed and hit the A&E ramp.

But on MAU, there was no hiding place. The furnace needed stoking twenty-four hours a day. Getting out of nights in the busiest department in the hospital was an absolute non-starter. So, I resigned myself to my fate. I was staring down the barrel of the 'rotational shift pattern.' It was a regime designed to dismantle your circadian rhythm with a sledgehammer. I prepared for the gruelling combination of days and nights, the limited family time, the death of my social life, and the inevitable cognitive decline where you lose the ability to distinguish between Tuesday morning and a fever dream.

The first couple of night shifts passed with a suspicious smoothness. It was a rhythm of routine maintenance: observations, fluid replenishments, PRN medications, and repositioning. Despite the metronomic beeping of the monitors and the dull hum of oxygen concentrators, the ward held a static atmosphere. It felt like a submarine running on silent.

How little I knew. This initial calm was luring me into a false sense of security. Here is a tip that might save your life: Never, and I mean never, use the 'Q' word out loud. Say the word 'quiet' and it is guaranteed that a patient who has been pleasant for three days will suddenly wake up as a delirious, villainous superhero. The problem was, nobody told me this until I leaned across the desk and sighed, 'God, this shift is on a go-slow. It's so... quiet.' I felt the glares of the staff burning my flesh. They looked at me as if I were the devil incarnate. And, right on cue, it began.

Little Mabel rose from her bed with wild hair and glazed eyes. There was a demonic quality to her movements. They were slow and methodical one moment, then jerky and uncontrolled. Mabel was independently mobile, so when she shuffled off, I assumed she was heading to the toilet. I sat silently (better than using the Q word) and kept her in my line of sight.

But Little Mabel didn't go to the toilet. She went hunting. She drifted over to Big Bert's bed, ripped down his blanket, and stared at his crotch with forensic intensity. The glaze in her eyes looked worryingly like excitement. I approached her slowly and whispered, 'Are you okay, Mabel?' She paused for seconds that felt like minutes. Finally, she looked at me and began to laugh hysterically. Then came the chanting. 'I only wanted to see his cock! I only wanted to see his cock!'

91

The shrill, rhythmic rendition of Mabel's new lyrics woke Big Bert from his slumber. If not for the absurdity, I would have been terrified. I never thought my sanity would be compromised by a 4ft 8", 92-year-old great-grandmother weighing less than 50kg. A few hours earlier, we had been crocheting baby hats for the neonatal unit while she told me about her great-grandchildren. Now, she was an agent of chaos. Her outburst destroyed the equilibrium, triggering a catastrophic domino effect that required an "all hands-on deck" response. And when I say all, I mean all. Security, porters, housekeeping. Anyone within earshot of the calamity was drafted in.

By this point, I had negotiated a fragile truce with the night shift. I was becoming confident in my rhythm. I understood that our role was not solely clinical care. It was crowd control. Our primary objective was to ensure calm prevailed until dawn with as little disruption as possible.

Then came the summons. It was a standard weekday night, around midnight, when my mentor dispatched an HCA to fetch me. I was to report to the nurses' station for a safety huddle. Now, safety huddles were a standard ritual. They usually happened around three hours into a shift. We stood in a circle and gave a breathless synopsis of every patient: presentation, diagnosis, treatment plan, and whatever investigation was currently blocking their discharge. The problem was, we had already done that. I walked down the corridor with a knot tightening in my stomach. I was unsure if we were having a second huddle for shits and giggles, or if I had personally cataclysmically screwed up. It didn't matter how experienced or confident I became. Every time a senior manager asked to see me, my internal monologue didn't whisper; it screamed. It was the primal, irrational certainty that the Regulator had finally noticed they'd made a clerical error in letting me in, and the police were on their way to confiscate my access card.

I arrived at the station expecting a reprimand. Instead, I walked into a funeral atmosphere. The mood was heavy. My mentor looked up from the computer screen, and, for the first time, I heard the words that every public-health employee dreads. 'Black Alert.' For the uninitiated, a 'Black Alert' was the nuclear option of hospital management. It signified that demand had not exceeded capacity; it had strangled it. It meant there were no beds, no trolleys, and likely no chairs left in the waiting room. Patient safety was compromised, and the system was effectively seizing. When a hospital declared this status, the drawbridge was pulled up. The A&E department was closed to incoming ambulances.

My mentor, a woman who usually possessed the blood pressure of a hibernating tortoise, looked oddly vibrationally stressed. A hive-like rash was creeping up her neck, and she was wringing her hands with the ferocity of attrition that threatened to spark a fire.

At first, I didn't understand the panic. In my naive, student brain, I did the maths. If the hospital was closed to trauma, surely that meant the tap was turned off. No more admissions. We could spend the night peacefully stabilising the current load and planning their imminent removal to the wards. Then the penny dropped. It hit the floor with the weight of an anvil. We weren't on Black Alert. Our nearest neighbour was. The shiny, state-of-the-art, flagship hospital had capitulated. They had closed their doors.

That meant every heart attack, stroke, car crash, and drunken brawl in a now more than double the size radius was being rerouted to us. We were the overflow drain for an entire Integrated Care System. Safety huddle over, my mentor grabbed me by the elbow. Her grip was a mix of maternal protection and military assertiveness. 'Cadet, take a twenty-minute break. Eat something. Drink plenty. Pee. Then report back to me. I'm going to need you tonight.'

There was a gravity in her voice that terrified me. But strangely, I also felt a surge of pride. I wasn't being sent to hide in the linen cupboard; I was being drafted. I did as I was told and stepped outside for a walk around the grounds. I inhaled the sharp, cold air, trying to mentally steel myself for the tsunami that was currently speeding down the arterial road towards us.

I circled around the block and approached the main entrance car park to find a strobe-light nightmare. It was a sea of pulsating blue. The sheer frequency of the flashing lights was enough to trigger a migraine, or perhaps a grand mal seizure even in the non-epileptic.

As I approached the sliding doors, I was intercepted. Some might describe it as accosted. A wall of high-vis jackets and Kevlar stepped in my path. It was security, looking less like hospital staff and more like nightclub bouncers bracing for a riot. He blocked the entrance, demanding I identify myself and my reasons for entering the fray.

I fumbled for my lanyard, flashing my student ID like a pathetic shield. Once entry was granted, I asked the gatekeeper what the situation was. He looked at me with the grim satisfaction of a disaster tourist. 'They're here already. We've got fourteen rigs stacked outside. Another nine are inbound. Dispatch says there are five holding in the field awaiting instruction.' The blood drained from my face. That wasn't a queue; it was a blockade. I didn't wait for further analysis. I turned and fast-walked back towards the MAU, my pace hovering on the edge of a sprint. Behind me, his voice boomed out like a doom-laden foghorn. 'Good luck, love. You're gonna need it.'

I returned to find my mentor assaulting the whiteboard. She was erasing patient details with the manic energy of a woman trying to destroy evidence. 'Rookie, you ready?' 'As I'll ever be,' I replied, checking my pockets for my pen torch and my sanity. 'Where do you need me?'
She outlined the battle plan. It was simple, desperate, and theoretically impossible. We were splitting every bed space in half to create a

conveyor belt system. One out, one up. We were to repeat this until the hospital capacity dropped below the critical threshold. 'Sounds like a plan,' I lied. 'What can I do?'

"I need you to complete all initial assessments and admission documentation on the new arrivals. Report anyone deteriorating. And Rookie? Don't let anyone die."

She handed me a walkie talkie, tuned to a private channel. It felt less like a clinical tool and more like a lifeline in a falling elevator. I clipped it to my belt and turned to head towards the double doors. "Rookie, where are you going?" she hollered. "To A&E," I shouted back. She looked at me like I was insane. "Fuck that. They're coming here. You need to triage in the corridor until the bed space is available." The only words my brain could formulate were, "Jesus Wept."

Anyone arriving on the unit had already been seen by a minimum of an F1, so the initial legwork was done. I began the relentless cycle of assessments, profiling their early warning scores to establish a baseline. In any normal situation, significant anomalies would be reported back to the admitting doctor immediately.

I was several patients deep into the corridor queue when I reached Carl. He was a mid-thirties male. According to his notes, he was an elite athlete, which meant his observations required a bit of context. A fitness fanatic of his calibre typically had a resting heart rate as low as forty something or fifty beats per minute. For most people, that level of bradycardia would mean they were nearing syncope or total unconsciousness, but for Carl, it was just a Tuesday.

I asked him how he was feeling. He was lucid and coherent, but he was sweating like a pig in a greenhouse. Then he said the next two words no nurse ever wants to hear. 'Chest pain.' I didn't reach for the obs machine. In an emergent situation, you never trust a machine if you are querying a result. I took his pulse manually. His heart rate was sitting in the high nineties and bounding. For a man whose heart usually ticked over like a luxury watch, this was a total system override.

A slow wave of panic began to creep in. I tried to compartmentalise my brain and run through my training. What next? I knew I needed to perform a full ABCDE assessment, but I made a split-second tactical decision to notify the clinician first. If the shit hit the fan and Carl went into cardiac arrest, I needed to know that help was already moving towards us.

Hobo, one of our regular repeat visitors, was sitting by the entrance of the bay. He went by that name because he lived in constant fear of being abducted by a higher power and refused to give his real name. This was despite it being printed on his hospital wristband in big, bold capital letters.

I approached him with a plan born of desperation. "Hobo, are you up for doing some security work for me?" "I'm, I'm, I'm good at that," he stuttered, before trailing off into a mumble about snipers and machine guns.

I moved him to the bay entrance and handed him his call bell. "Right, Hobo. Do you see this man here?" I pointed animatedly at Carl. "Don't take your eyes off him. Do you understand?" "Yes ma'am," Hobo replied, snapping to attention. "If he looks any different to how he looks now, and I mean any different, you ring this bell. But Hobo, this is a top-secret mission. Don't tap it like you do when you want a tea. Press it hard and hold it down. You got it?" "Yes ma'am."

Holding a call bell down triggers the emergency alarm. It usually signifies one of two things: cardiac arrest or respiratory failure. It causes every resuscitation-trained team member on the ward to descend instantly. They arrive like a flock of crows circling fresh roadkill. I turned to Carl, reassured him, and told him to signal Hobo if he felt himself slipping.

In hindsight, this was a spectacular error in judgment. I should never have taught Hobo the power of the hold down. For the rest of his stay, he triggered the emergency alarm at sporadic times of the day to time the response. He recorded the results in a pocket notebook and ran a sweepstake with the other patients, trading biscuits, jelly, and ice cream based on the ward's performance.

You are not allowed to run in a hospital, even in the most dire emergencies. It creates panic and, more practically, you're likely to collide with a trolley or a precarious drip stand. Instead, I walked with extreme purpose toward the doctors' office at the end of the corridor. I burst through the door. No doctors. I grabbed my walkie-talkie, with sweat in my hand. "Where are the doctors? I have an emergent patient. I need an assessment, stat." The reply came back through a wall of static. My mentor voice sounded weary. "Fat chance. They've all been deployed to the rigs. They're triaging in situ to try and avoid admissions."

I stood in the empty office, listening to the hum of the computers. It was a perverse paradox. I was in a hospital specifically designed for emergency intake, yet it was currently devoid of a single available doctor. Great.

I frog-marched myself back toward the bay, switching the walkie talkie to channel two. I radioed the Rapid Response Team and put them on standby. On the way, I spotted a rare and highly sought-after prize: an abandoned ECG machine. I half-inched it immediately, navigating the device through a corridor that was rapidly becoming a graveyard of trolleys and acutely unwell patients.

Back at the watchtower, Hobo hadn't moved an inch. He held his call bell with the white-knuckled grip of an assassin waiting for the green light. Carl was sitting upright, a ghost of colour returning to his cheeks. "How are you feeling?" "A little better," he rasped.

I gained consent for the tests and began the ABCDE assessment. Usually, I would talk a patient through every step, but time was a luxury I didn't have. I worked in relative silence, the only sound being the Velcro of the BP cuff and the whirring of the ECG as it began churning out paper like a 1980s fax machine.

I was no cardiologist, but even I could see the readout was a disaster. Instead of a uniform row of peaks and troughs, the paper showed a jagged, frantic derangement. I walked with extreme purpose to the nearest phone and dialled the emergency number.

Within seconds, we were shrouded. A gowned-up phalanx of specialists, advanced clinicians, and resus-trained nurses descended, bringing enough equipment to perform surgery in a field. While the team lead spoke to Carl, who remained eerily coherent, I handed over the early warning score and the ECG strip.

Bowed heads. Hushed whispers. The term 'acute infarct' was tossed around like a live grenade. The senior clinician turned to Carl. "Sir, you are having a heart attack. We need to get you to A&E. Now"

Before the sentence had even finished, the bed was lowered into the supine position, the pads were in situ, and Carl was being rocketed down the corridor. The Doctor looked back at me for a split second. "Good spot!" My mentor appeared through the chaos. "What happened?" I replied, "He didn't die."

The aftermath felt like the centre of a cyclone. It was eerily still, yet my body was internally humming from the urgency. I took two seconds to breathe, then I turned to the next patient in the queue.

I moved from one patient to the next, then on to the next, until the triage of the overflow was as up to date as it could possibly be. I searched out my mentor and asked what was next. She had allocated the other student nurse, Immi, to facilitate transfers and discharges alongside the flow team. The backlog was clearing, and there were dozens of patients ready to be moved. "The porters are slammed," my mentor said. "Team up with Immi and start transferring patients to their scheduled wards."

Later, following this experience, I requested a spoke placement with the operations hub. It was a revelation. Looking at the admissions and discharge boards was like standing on the floor of a Las Vegas casino. I was staring at a hundred spinning slot machine wheels, and the only way to stop them was to find a patient a non-existent bed. The pressure was atmospheric. Did I want to work in operations? Fuck no.

We quickly computed that we needed to flip the entire ward. That meant four bays of six patients each had to be decanted to other areas of the hospital or moved to the discharge hub. Naturally, the hub was inconveniently housed at the exact opposite end of the building from MAU. It felt like we were running a marathon in paper-thin shoes.

By the time the penultimate patient was transferred, Immi and I were strolling back to the ward at a significantly slower pace. We were starting to feel the burn in our calves and the gritty sting of exhaustion in our eyes.

Immi, who was very fitness conscious taught me a trick. As nurses we are prohibited from wearing jewellery other than stud earrings and one plain band. We also had to be bare below the elbows, so no watches, bracelets of those charity band things. She taught me to put my Fitbit on my ankle so I could still track my steps. Not that bothered I asked why she did it and her reply was that the more steps she did at work, the less she had to do in the gym. Fair point. Glad I had that night though; I'd cracked up 24,000 steps. In my book that equated to 24,000 steps I didn't need to take in my non-existent exercise regime. I concluded that if every step amounted to one minute of binge-watching Netflix, I had 400 hours' worth in the bank.

We arrived back to find a spread of posh coffees and pastries from Costa, courtesy of the Ward Manager. We stood there, blinking at the caffeine like it was a mirage. "Are we thinking the same thing'" I asked. Immi nodded slowly. "I think so. What the hell is the Ward Manager doing here? And why on earth is the coffee shop open?" We looked at our fob watches, and the revelation hit us like a physical weight. It was after nine. We hadn't just finished a shift; we had survived a siege and worked two hours into the next morning without even noticing.

My mentor bounded over, looking remarkably fresh compared to our bedraggled states. "Thanks for staying on, guys. You properly proved yourselves last night. Job well done!" Up until that second, I had been operating on pure autopilot, a machine fuelled by cortisol and clinical necessity. Now, the battery was dead. I could suddenly feel every movement of my joints, the shallow rasp of every breath, and the agonising weight of every step.

I checked my phone and saw that The Boy had dutifully checked in at school. With the maternal panic subsided, I called a dear friend. I called her Mumma Bear. She also worked at the hospital and lived a short distance away. When she picked up, she practically squealed down the line. "Shit, chick! I heard about last night. Are you still alive?" "Barely," I replied. I was speaking monosyllabically because I couldn't fathom the energy required to formulate a full sentence. My brain felt like a browser with too many tabs open, all of them frozen.

"Hold fire," she said, her voice shifting into a commanding, protective tone. "I'll come and pick you up. You can crash at mine after a hot bath." I closed my eyes for a second, leaning on the cold hospital brickwork. I love that woman to absolute pieces.

This placement taught me the exigency of decompression. The art of it, however, remained a work in progress. Some shifts hit harder than others. They were all busy, but some were on the verge of manic. There were shifts that were purely physically exhausting, and then there were those that were emotionally draining, leaving your sympathy tank bone-dry. The ones I struggled to unwind from were the ones that were both. The Black Alert night was the latter.

Cocooned in my mate's spare bed, with her dog, Charlie Pig, and two cats, Blue and Lucy, for company, I desperately tried to shut down. I tried to block out the visual flashbacks, the echo of the bells, the rhythmic chirp of the monitors, and the sound of patients wailing in pain. But as the external sounds faded and my muscles finally began to slacken, the inevitable happened. Thought encroached.

That last early warning score I recorded was a three; did I escalate it? If I did, who to? Did I pack that man's inhaler when he was transferred, or was it still lying on the bedside table? Did I phone that woman's husband to tell him she'd been moved? I say 'her' and 'him' because, by this point, I couldn't remember a single name. I had a blurry mental gallery of faces and bed spaces. Or where I thought the bed spaces were.

The feeling of dread before your next shift was palpable. It was a cold, heavy weight in the pit of your stomach. The fear that you overlooked something, missed a subtle sign, or inadvertently caused harm is an element of nursing you never truly shake.

If you are going to survive this career, you need to find your coping strategies. You need them to steer clear of the burnout that waits for every nurse who carries the whole hospital home with them. I arrived for my next shift with a tight, cold knot in my stomach. Everyone from the Black Alert night had been called into a debrief session. These meetings were designed to dissect the effectiveness of emergency protocols, what went right, what went wrong, and how the system buckled. They generally went one of two ways. You were either praised for your responsiveness and performance, or you were given a royal bollocking and told to do better.

Surprisingly, it was the former. We were commended for our grit under pressure. We all left the room feeling relatively unscathed and ready for a standard day's work. However, that feeling was short-lived.

As the group dispersed, my mentor and I were singled out and summoned to the conference room to meet with the shift lead. This was no longer a team debrief; this was a targeted meeting. My mind immediately raced back to every chart I'd signed and every patient I'd triaged in that dark corridor.

On the way down the hall, I leaned in and whispered to my mentor, "Do I need to be worried?" A woman of few words and even fewer pretences, she didn't offer any hollow comfort. She looked straight ahead and replied, "Fucked if I know."

On arrival we were acknowledged, rather than greeted, by a member of the HR team who ushered us to two seats positioned side by side. The problem was that the seats were on the wrong side of an extremely long, wide table. It gave off what I imagined were very important prejudicial congress vibes.

After an agonising wait, the door opened. Two unidentified suits, the Chief Nurse, the A&E Ward Manager and our shift lead walked in.

They moved in a single, silent line, like some sort of military parade. I wasn't sure whether I was supposed to rise to the occasion and take an oath or sit there and fake a sense of calm.

My mentor sat staunchly upright in her chair. She possessed a legendary stiff upper lip and didn't move a single muscle. I followed suit, bracing myself to run the crucible with her by my side.

The Chief Nurse didn't waste any time with pleasantries. The upshot was that it had been brought to the board's attention that I, a mere Student Nurse, had been the one responsible for triggering the 2222 Rapid Response Team.

In the hierarchy of a hospital, that is a significant trigger to pull. The 2222 bleep is the "break glass in case of emergency" button for the entire facility. It isn't just a phone call. It is an activation of high-level resources that costs thousands of pounds in man-hours and diverts the most senior clinicians in the building away from their current tasks. For a student to bypass the chain of command and initiate that response is, to put it mildly, unconventional.

The room was silent. I could feel the weight of the collective gaze of the hospital's elite. I waited for the hammer to fall. A loaded pause prevailed while we waited for some sort of question or further explanation. My mentor eventually broke the silence. Her tone was calm, though clearly tinged with incredulity. "That is correct," she said. The Chief Nurse leaned forward. "In line with emergency protocol, student nurses are not permitted to lone work without the direct supervision of their mentor."

During yet another weighted juncture, I could see the frustration building in my mentor posture. "Student Nurse Victoria is a highly capable and valued member of the team. She has demonstrated the ability to perform routine tasks efficiently and accurately, even in the direst of situations. I asked nothing more of her than I would from an experienced healthcare assistant, a role she also held prior to her training. I assessed her competency routinely throughout the shift and had no concerns regarding her performance or her competency to practice the clinical tasks I had assigned."

One of the unidentified suits practically bellowed his response. "This still doesn't explain the unauthorised use of the 2222 bleep without instruction from a registered clinician though, does it?" My mentor didn't blink. "No. It does not. Perhaps you should ask the man whose life she saved what he thinks?"

The air went out of the room. After a great deal of huffing, puffing, and hushed whispers among the right side of the table, a boring, monosyllabic rendition of the emergency protocol was recited to us. We were dismissed.

Before we reached the door, my mentor turned back to the panel. "Out of curiosity, can I ask who notified you of this matter? It would be in my interest to know so that I can provide some further training and mentorship for them regarding emergency protocol."

Despite being strictly prohibited from sharing that information, the Ward Manager blurted out, "Oh, it was another student. She wanted to know why she didn't get to trigger the 2222." God, give me strength.

Immi and I didn't share any more conversations about Fitbits or other equally unimportant things. In a world of Black Alerts and life-or-death decisions, I realised that some people are more interested in the drama of the alarm than the pulse of the patient.

The day of my final assessment arrived. As I have already made clear, my mentor was driven, focused, and until you truly got to know her, could come across as giving everyone short shrift. She didn't believe in grand ceremonies or long-winded farewells. She simply handed me my assessment folder. "Right, Victoria, here you are. It's self-explanatory, so I'll leave this with you. If you need anything added, find me before you leave your last shift."

I took the folder and found a quiet corner to open it. I glanced at the final score. Ninety-five. I looked up to find her watching me from across the ward. "You should have got full marks," she said, her voice carrying over the hum of a nebuliser. "But I'm damned if I'm being moderated by the Uni for over-grading again."

I couldn't help but laugh. I had survived a Black Alert, triaged an entire corridor, and saved a man's life, only to be hauled before a board of suits for unauthorised excellence. Now, I was being marked down slightly simply to avoid a paperwork headache for the department.

I walked out of the hospital and into the crisp morning air, feeling the familiar internal hum of a long shift. I was leaving the unit with tens of thousands of steps on my clock, a solid grade in my folder, and the knowledge that when a patient was dying in front your very eyes it was best practice to find someone else to bleep 2222. Reprimanded or not, moderated or not, I was nearly a nurse. And the kind of nurse the suits couldn't handle but the patients desperately needed.

So that was it. MAU was done. I felt strangely broken yet enlivened, shellshocked but accomplished. The positives certainly outweighed the negatives, but the negatives were low, so very low. This wasn't because of the patients, the acuteness of their illnesses, or the very real pressures of caring for people in their most fragile states. It was the work culture.

This environment had a different kind of energy, perhaps because it was so fast paced. What I noticed most was the culture of placing blame, pointing fingers, and the constant reporting of minor human error. Maybe I was a little jaded before starting there because MAU certainly had a reputation that preceded the vital work they did there every single day.

Funnily enough, by the end of my placement, MAU had been turned into AMU. Reorganising the initials in the name of a ward would clearly result in a department transitioning into a well led and safe environment overnight. Just because it was called something marginally different did not eradicate or detract from the fact that this particular unit had a toxic reputation with an ingrained bullying and blame culture.

The ward management spent more time fighting abuse claims than they did coordinating the treatment of patients. These claims were by nurses, about nurses. The patients, ironically, were fine and dandy. They were as happy as pigs in shit, blissfully unaware of the civil war happening behind the nursing station.

07

How to Be a Student Nurse and

Survive the Institutional Silence

There is a peculiar, physiological glitch in the human condition that I have never quite been able to map. I cannot fathom how the body manages to process exhaustion with the exact same severity, regardless of the cause. Whether you have survived a twelve-hour "critical" night shift, fuelled by cortisol and the fear of God, or you have simply endured six hours of back-to-back lecture theatre sessions on public health policy, the physical result is identical. Your bones ache, your eyelids feel like they have been weighted with lead shot, and your brain turns into a stagnant pond. This day was no exception. The only difference was that instead of dodging cardiac arrests, I was trapped in an afternoon of Evidence Based Learning.

This session was billed as "relatively non-interactive," which is academic code for "sit there and listen while I read a PowerPoint to you." We were being presented with our next case study, a thrill ride that promised to be as engaging as watching paint dry in a humidity chamber. However, the facilitator had a trick up their sleeve. The highlight of the day, arguably the highlight of the entire block so far, was their decision to reallocate the group members.

It felt exactly like that pivotal, sadistic moment in *The Apprentice*, right before the interviews. It is the moment where the boss decides to shuffle the teams, not because it makes logical business sense, but to see how the candidates cope when their support structures are obilterated. Or, more likely, to incite conflict, exacerbate volatility, and ensure the viewing figures spike for the broadcaster. I had spent months moulding and nurturing my previous team. We were a well-oiled machine, a catalyst for high grades and low stress. We were moments away from victory. And then, at the final hurdle, my key players were snatched away. In their place, I was left staring at a defunct group of individuals whose previous academic performances had done little to inspire confidence. These were people whose "product or service" I wouldn't buy at a car boot sale, let alone invest my degree in.

With the team member introductions complete, we siphoned off into our respective groups. We briefly discussed the case presentation, allocated roles and responsibilities, and headed home. The session was meant to last under two hours, but the facilitator practically had their car running before we had left the room. We safely assumed it was acceptable to go AWOL.

On reflection and taking into consideration the past performances of the new group members, I began to feel marginally more positive. As I planned the structure of the presentation, I allocated who would be best for each role. I had already self-appointed myself as group and presentation coordinator. The others didn't know it yet, but I was sure they wouldn't mind.

In my group sat Mr Z, a person with a surname that strongly resembled a common household implement. I use the word 'man' deliberately. He was the only other student in our cluster born before 1992. He had no social media presence to speak of, and when questioned in class, he didn't stutter; he responded by quoting an article written by a scholarly genius.

Until that day, however, we had never spoken. You would assume that the two most vintage students in the room would naturally gravitate towards each other, bonding over our shared antiquity. Not in this instance. Mr Z was a Mental Health student.

Even in nursing, basic human and social instinct prevails. Mental Health nurses stick with Mental Health nurses. Children's nurses stick with Children's nurses. The only deviation from this segregation was us. Adult nurses pick up the fodder. We look after anyone and everyone. We have the ability to infiltrate each speciality group should we so wish, but we also attract the strays because we know a little bit about everything. Some call us a jack of all trades, master of none. I prefer to think of us as widely researched and infinitely capable.

The following week of EBL went as well as could be expected, which is to say it was a slow march towards the inevitable. We laid out the fruits of our research and highlighted the key points. Then we hit the wall: how to deliver a message so banal it threatened to sedate us all, whilst somehow making it "engaging and thought-provoking."

The awkward silence was too much to bear. It was the sort of quiet where you can hear the fluorescent lights humming. I decided to break it. I asked the group if anyone would like to be appointed group coordinator.

Tumbleweed.

I pivoted to strategy. I pointed out that this was a golden opportunity for one of them. Leading the group meant gaining reviews and testimonies from the rest of us, perfect evidence for the participation section of our Practice Assessment Portfolios. Nursing students usually hunt for portfolio evidence like it is sustenance, so I waited for the bite.

More tumbleweed.

Finally, the quietest student in the group looked up from their notebook. They tentatively whispered, "Victoria, would you like to do it?" "Sure thing," I replied. I kept the triumph out of my voice. That was settled. A touch of reverse psychology had worked wonders. I had the role I wanted, and they thought they were doing me a favour.

I am a "go hard or go home" sort of person. Though, truthfully, at this stage in my life, going home is usually the more appealing of the two options. I am a marginally older student and bring with that a level of resilience purely as a result of hard life experiences. I don't do half measures. I immediately set about planning a method of delivery that was interactive, current, and aggressively topical. I wanted to present without presenting.

If anyone so much as utters the word "PowerPoint" to me, I involuntarily recoil. I slip into a catatonic state where the lights are technically on, but the house has been repossessed. Death by PowerPoint is a genuine clinical risk as far as I am concerned, and I refused to inflict it on the class.

If you have the dubious pleasure of meeting anyone I have worked with in this capacity, they will likely describe my approach as "off the wall." They might even use words like "questionable" or "controversial." I take these as compliments. I have a reputation for delivering information in a way that ensures you cannot ignore it, even if you want to. This case study was to be no exception.

The patient in this case study immediately reminded me of a book I had read that was subsequently adapted into a major motion picture: *The Diving Bell and the Butterfly* by Jean-Dominique Bauby.

I strongly urge you to both read the book and watch the film. Not necessarily in that order. You won't fully appreciate one without the other, so make sure you do both at some point. The effect this book and its enlightening cinematography had on me was profound. Rarely does a "story" impact me emotionally to the point where I actively, and quite literally, alter my working practices. But this did.

I am so fortunate to have discovered it early in my healthcare career. When I say discovered, I really mean it was recommended and given to me by a fellow colleague. They were one of the most caring, pure, and accepting individuals I have ever worked with. They have since become a dear friend.

I am going to dance around the specifics here. I need to convey the essence of this concept without ruining the discovery. I want you to stumble upon the captivating, awe-inspiring character of this narrative without any preconception or influence, as I did. Consider this a deliberate narrative redaction.

So, for the purposes of this explanation, all I will tell you is that we utilised a chapter of the book entitled "The Wheelchair." It was a short, descriptive piece. A little under seven hundred words. Three minutes of spoken word. In the context of a seminar room, three minutes usually feels like a lifetime, but we needed every second.

My aim was to move beyond the usual "death by PowerPoint" apathy. Well, let's call it our aim, once I had informed the group of what we were doing and they had wisely agreed. I didn't want to tell the audience how a patient might feel. I wanted to show them. I wanted to force a palpable experience upon them.

We planned to take turns reading the passage. We would strip away the usual mumbled, rushed delivery of tremulous students and replace it with a slow, deliberate cadence. We would use as much emphasis as we could muster. And whilst we read, we would introduce the "palpable experience" via total immersion. We were going to make them feel it.

Prior to the reading, I stepped forward to introduce our "case study." I didn't want them passively listening; I wanted them physically and emotionally engaged. I asked them, provided they felt comfortable, to extend both arms out at length in front of them and close their eyes. It sounded like the beginning of a dubious hypnosis act or a cult induction, but to my surprise, everyone complied. A sea of arms shot out. Eyelids fluttered shut. Perfect. The first hurdle was cleared without anyone laughing in my face.

I delivered the disclaimer with the tone of a flight attendant pointing out the emergency exits. I explained that if, at any point, they felt the slightest discomfort, or if their focus began to drift from the spoken words, they should immediately lower their arms or open their eyes.

I emphasized that the most important element of this exercise was their comfort. There was no judgement here. The primary objective was the absorption of the text, and whatever their body needed to do to achieve that was valid. There was no right or wrong way to be a human in this room. Do as your mind and body dictate.

Internally, however, I knew this could go one of two ways. It would either be a profound educational moment, or a cringe-inducing disaster that I would relive every night before sleep for the next decade. I had beta-tested the concept on The Boy at home. At the time he possessed the concentration span of a peanut, yet even he had stilled during the test run. I figured that if a room full of nursing students possessed at least the same cognitive baseline as my teenager, we might actually pull this off.

One by one, my group members picked up the narrative baton, reading their allocated sections with the slow, deliberate pacing we had rehearsed. The room was still, save for the collective breath of thirty people holding a static pose.

Within seconds, the physiology kicked in. Lactic acid is a powerful persuasion tool. A couple of the students lowered their arms almost immediately, their deltoids surrendering to the burn. Then came the domino effect. Some opened their eyes, presumably to check if they were the only ones failing. Upon seeing that their peers had also lowered their arms, the social contract of the exercise shattered. They either gritted their teeth in determined martyrdom or allowed their limbs to drop with a sigh of relief.

As we drew to the end of the second minute, the room was a landscape of defeat. All but one participant had lowered their arms, and about half had opened their eyes. Their focus had shifted from the tragic narrative to their own physical discomfort.

By the end of the third minute, the surrender was total, bar one. All arms were down. Only a smattering of people remained with their eyes closed, still desperately trying to absorb the information through the haze of distraction.

On completion, we allowed the silence to hang in the air. We held a dramatic pause, letting the weight of the moment settle before inviting everyone to make themselves comfortable. I nodded specifically to the one person who had looked like a statue, arms stretched an eyes tightly shut for the full duration.

We took a moment to process the scene before opening the floor to discussion. The silence was absolute. You could have heard a pin drop.

We broke the silence by declaring the room a designated safe space. We invited them to perform an autopsy on their own reactions during the exercise. I wanted to know everything. I wanted the physical complaints about the lactic burn in their shoulders. I wanted the psychological anxiety of the self-imposed blindness. I wanted the raw emotional response to the tragedy we had read aloud.

This was a free exchange. The floor was open for anything and everything they had felt, endured, or suppressed in the last three minutes.

The response was eye-opening. For some, it was literally eye-watering. The stoicism of the nursing student usually runs deep, but the dam broke. Several students were shedding tears, their composure fracturing as they tried to articulate how the words of the passage had landed.

The adjectives started flying around the room like shrapnel. "Debilitated." "Unheard." "Isolated." "Helpless." "Frustrated."

This list was not exhaustive, but it was heavy. These weren't just buzzwords to be written in a reflective essay; they were feelings that were actively suffocating the room. We had stripped away the clinical distance and left them with the raw, uncomfortable reality of the patient experience.

As the emotional dust settled, I moved to close the presentation. I turned my attention to the only person in the room who had desperately hung onto the physical element of the task until the bitter end. It was our facilitator. She sat there, looking rather pleased with her display of stamina.

I addressed her directly. I asked them, quite simply, how the content of the passage had made her feel. I asked what specific emotions the narrative had stirred in her.

She blinked. The silence stretched.

She couldn't answer. She hadn't heard a word.

She had been too consumed by the burn in their shoulders to process the story. She was so focused on winning the "keep your arms up and eyes closed" competition, she had spent the last three minutes battling her own physiology to prove a point. In doing so, they had rendered themselves deaf to the patient's voice. It was a perfect, accidental metaphor for modern healthcare. She had followed the rules perfectly and missed the point entirely.

The presentation concluded. The feedback was outstanding. We swept the board, scoring a "high" in every single category. We had turned a classroom into an empathy chamber and survived.

Feeling a surge of pride, and with The Boy out for the night, I retreated to the sanctuary of my living room. I slipped into a onesie. It was the uniform of the off-duty, exhausted mother: less fashion statement, more mummified surrender. I poured a glass of cider from a plastic large bottle. In a different life, or perhaps a solvency-adjacent one, it would have been a heavy Malbec from a bottle with a cork. But I am a skint, middle-aged student. The grapes of wrath come in plastic now.

I sat down and hit play on the film that had secured our academic victory. I watched *The Diving Bell and the Butterfly* alone in the dark.

And I cried. Hard.

It wasn't a cinematic, single-tear sort of cry. It was ugly. I am not sure if the trigger was the film itself, or if the narrative just cracked the seal on a pressurised tank of other things. Exhaustion. Loneliness. Crippling financial hardship. General, pervasive discontentment. They all poured out at once.

I decided not to analyse it. That way madness lies. Instead, I wiped my face, turned off the TV, and went to bed. I have a very large, imaginary magic rug in my head. Over the years, I have become remarkably adept at sweeping such emotions underneath it, leaving the floorboards clear for the next day's crisis.

I was tucked up in bed, hovering in that narcotic sweet spot between consciousness and coma. It is that heavy, warm paralysis where you are not quite asleep, but you are blissfully aware that you are nearly there. It is the best feeling in the world.

Then, the room bleached white for a split second. A loud ping cut through the silence.

My flat was effectively a walk-in fridge. The gas and electric meters were engaged in a starvation contest, running on fumes and prayer. The rule was simple: if The Boy wasn't home, the heating stayed off. I was essentially preserving myself in cryostasis to save loose change.

I didn't want to move. I certainly didn't want to reach for my phone. To do so would break the hermetic seal of the duvet I had expertly wrapped around myself, allowing the sub-zero air to seep in. I ran the calculus. It was a little after midnight. No one, and I mean absolutely no one in my life, would attempt to contact me at such an unearthly hour. My social life was dead, and work or university administration usually waited until morning to ruin my day.

After some mental deliberation, I realised there was a slight statistical possibility it might be The Boy. It was highly unlikely, but conceivable, nonetheless. Maternal duty overrides biological preservation every time.

I tried to minimize the damage. I reached one arm out, keeping the rest of me buried, and began tapping my bedside table blindly. I was trying to locate the phone by touch alone. The attempt was futile.

I had to commit. I sat up. The air hit me like a physical slap. I could see my own breath pluming in the darkness as I exhaled. I snapped the lamp on, grabbed the glowing source of the disturbance, and retreated instantly to my haven. I pulled the covers over my head, creating a warm, breath-filled tent, trying to restore my body temperature to something compatible with life before checking the screen.

I squinted at the screen, one eye squeezed shut to block the sudden glare. I opened WhatsApp to a message from the digital void. "Hi, hope you don't mind, I wanted to say thanks for your input with the presentation, I thought it went really well."

I had absolutely no idea who this was. The sender was a ghost, identified only by a string of random digits. I knew it was one of the EBL group members, as we had reluctantly exchanged numbers for the sole purpose of coordinating the presentation. However, I operate on a strict "need to know" basis. I hadn't saved any of them to my contacts. To me, they were data points in a temporary group chat.

Still half-asleep, and lacking the cognitive bandwidth for detective work, I typed out a generic, diplomatic reflex. "No problem, I think so too, great to work with you all." I dropped the phone, snuggled back down into my thermal cocoon, and drifted back towards the precipice of sleep. I dreamt of dreaming.

About twenty minutes passed. I was settling into the warmth when the room was violated for a second time.

Ping.

I groaned. I fished the phone back out.

"Do you mind if I share something with you?"

I stared at the screen. I still had no idea who I was talking to. But now, the irritation was mixed with intrigue. Who from the EBL group would be messaging me at stupid o'clock with such a loaded question? It sounded like the precursor to a confession, or perhaps a pyramid scheme pitch.

Curiosity is a dangerous flaw in a nurse, but it is a dominant one. I typed a single word.

"Sure."

I waited. The typing bubble appeared. Then the message landed.

Oh my. Oh my. Oh my.

And there it was. In all its graphic, high-definition glory.

My body reacted before my brain had even finished downloading the visual data. It was a pure, spinal reflex. A gut reaction kicked in, bypassing all logic. I slammed the home button to kill the light, erupted from my thermal cocoon, and propelled the phone across the room. I didn't just drop it. I jettisoned it as if the casing had suddenly become radioactive. It clattered against the far wall and landed in the darkness.

It was the exact same physiological recoil you experience when someone sends you one of those internet "screamer" videos. You know the ones. You stare intently at a serene landscape for ten seconds, and then a decomposing face screams at you at full volume. You lose your composure. You lose your dignity. You lose your shit.

I sat bolt upright in bed, hyperventilating in the freezing air. The cold didn't matter anymore. My heart was hammering my ribs like a trapped bird. I stared at the corner where the device lay dormant.

"What the actual fuck!?!"

It did not require the deductive powers of a seasoned investigator to solve the mystery. My brain rebooted. I desperately tried to process the limited data available to me while sitting in the freezing dark.

The demographics of our EBL group were stark. It was a hen house with only a few foxes. As one of less than 30% males in our cohort, the suspect list had a population of not many.

The man with the household surname. The vintage scholar. The Mental Health nurse who quoted academic journals and didn't have a social media profile. Apparently, the lack of social media presence was not due to a desire for privacy, but perhaps to avoid a digital paper trail for this sort of behaviour.

The question that screamed through my mind was not who, but why. Why, in the name of all things holy, had this person sent me a photo of their erect cock?

I genuinely didn't know what to think, let alone what to do. My processing skills had crashed. My operating system was devoid of all function, leaving my body numb. The single word "Why" circled around my head like a buffering icon that refused to load.

If I wasn't awake before, I was certainly awake now. I sat up for hours, staring into the gloom. Eventually, I mustered the courage to crawl across the freezing floor and check the message. I had to be sure. I needed to rule out a night terror, a fever dream, or a carbon monoxide-induced hallucination.

I looked. It was still there. It was very much still there.

I deliberated for the rest of the night, running scenarios until the early hours of the morning. Eventually, I drifted off into a sleep that was far from restful.

Then came the morning. You know that feeling. That split second of bliss when you wake up and the slate is clean. You stretch, you yawn, and the world is fine. And then, boom. You get hit by the events you have desperately tried to forget. It is a cortisol hangover.

My magic rug was not working that day. The lump underneath it was too big to ignore.

I spent the morning swinging wildly between options. Do I ignore it? Do I report them? Was it a joke? What on earth did they expect me to do with this information?

I still, to this day, do not know why I decided on my course of action. Perhaps my brain had simply snapped under the pressure. But flippantly, and true to form, I decided to go down the humorous route. Humour is the only weapon I know how to wield effectively. I refused to be a victim; I would make them a joke.

I typed two words.

"Ding Dong."

I followed it with an unhealthy amount of crying-laughing emojis.

The three dots of doom danced on the screen for what felt like an eternity. Then, the reply landed.

"Why are you laughing, are you not impressed?"
It is notoriously difficult to decipher emotional nuance via text message, yet somehow, the tone was unmistakable. They sounded positively disappointed. They sounded hurt.

Them? Hurt? The audacity was breathless.

I stared at the phone in disbelief. They had sent an unsolicited, graphic image of their anatomy to a fellow student in the middle of the night, and their primary concern was that I wasn't offering a standing ovation.

They clearly didn't understand the taxonomy of my laughter. They assumed I was reviewing the dimensions of their body like a critic at an art gallery. They failed to grasp that my reaction had nothing to do with size and everything to do with the situation. It wasn't a giggle of ridicule; it was the hysterical, high-pitched screech of "what the actual fuck are you doing?"

The absurdity of their wounded pride finally shocked my brain back into gear. I rediscovered my faculties. I realised that engaging with this level of delusion was above my pay grade.

I decided to implement a full communications embargo. I would absolutely not respond, under any circumstances.

The subsequent weeks at university were an exercise in tactical evasion. They were indescribably awkward, emotionally draining, and simply unenjoyable. I spent less time focusing on the course content and more time scanning corridors like a bodyguard expecting an assassination attempt.

Fortunately, the academic structure provided some natural fortification. If it was Mr Z, he and I were studying separate disciplines so our paths only crossed during the core foundation teaching hall sessions. These were held in the main theatres, vast caverns filled with a cohort over two hundred strong. I used the sheer volume of bodies to my advantage. I treated my fellow students as human shields, burying myself in the middle of the pack, far away from the peripheral vision of the person who had overshared so spectacularly.

On the rare occasions where our orbits did collide, I abandoned all social grace. I didn't feign blindness or pretend to check my phone. I unapologetically turned one hundred and eighty degrees and walked in the opposite direction. My refusal to engage was absolute. The message was clear: the treaty of friendship was burned. Eye contact and pleasantries were a thing of the past.

I assumed the radio silence meant they had finally understood the gravity of their error. I assumed they were wallowing in shame.
I was wrong.

As my heart rate was returning to a resting rhythm, the phone buzzed. They had messaged.

It was an attempt at an apology. I think. In the same way that a hit-and-run driver reversing over the victim to check for damage is an "attempt" at first aid. It wasn't heartfelt. It was barely coherent. Depending on your interpretation of the English language, it was borderline accusatory.

The narrative they spun was that they were "struggling" in their relationship. They explained, with zero self-awareness, that they had sent the graphic, unsolicited image as an outlet for their pent-up sexual frustration.

My brain stuttered. Their WHAT?

The revelation hit me like a wet fish. It turned out this person wasn't just a creep; they were a committed creep. They were newly partnered. They had a young family at home. Yet, they felt their predatory behaviour justified because of a lack of sexual fulfilment: that their partner who was likely exhausted raising their children wasn't providing.

They had decided to outsource their domestic dissatisfaction to my phone. It was a monologue of self-pity. It was an explanation with absolutely no regard for how their "outlet" might have impacted me. I scanned the text three times, hunting for the word "sorry." It was most definitely not present. They weren't apologising for the act; they were explaining why they were the real victim.

I did mention they were studying Mental Health nursing, right? The irony was so dense it was practically choking me. Here was a person training to support the vulnerable minds of others, yet they possessed the emotional intelligence of a brick.

Despite the absolute communication vacuum from my end, the messages continued to arrive with the sporadic unpredictability of an AF heart rhythm. Over the next few weeks, I became an unwilling receptacle for their consciousness. It was as if I had been conscripted as their virtual, pro bono therapist, a safe space for them to vent their innermost thoughts and feelings without the inconvenience of a bill.

Then, I broke my cardinal rule.

It was baffling. It was as if I had been subliminally brainwashed. I appeared to have developed a digital strain of Stockholm Syndrome, even though I was clinically aware of exactly what that was and how stupid I was being. Against all better judgement, I felt a twinge of professional pity for him.

Now, let's put this into the context of studying nursing. It turns out that the conditioning works. All those mundane sessions we had endured, the ones where we stared at slide after slide of PowerPoints while the facilitator droned on about 'holistic care,' had finally permeated my skull. They had drilled into my psyche the need to channel compassion and empathy, even when the patient is repelling you.

The programming finally kicked in. I decided to try and help him.

My motivation was a complex cocktail. Part of it was a genuine, albeit reluctant, desire to help a drowning man save his soul. But the other part was risk management. I wanted to highlight that this behaviour was pathological. I needed to show them that this wasn't healthy, in the hope that I could prevent them from inflicting this on anyone else.

Lord knows, I didn't want another woman to feel the way I did. I was attempting to triage the situation before they created more casualties.

It began as an exercise in genuine professional concern. I approached it like a triage nurse handling a difficult walk-in. I advised them. I signposted them towards legitimate support networks. I made it abundantly clear that they needed to speak to their partner, a trusted confidant, or a paid professional. I clarified, repeatedly, that I fell into none of those categories. I was a student nurse trying to keep my own head above water, not a life raft for a submerging adulterer.

However, the more I engaged, the more the depth of their narcissism revealed itself. It leaked from every message like an infected wound.

It wasn't the self-indulgent content of their texts that gave them away; it was the structure of the dialogue. Or rather, the monologue. In all those weeks of digital vomiting, they never once asked about me. Not a single question.

They didn't ask if I was okay. They didn't ask about my life, my family, or my own struggles. To them, I wasn't a person. I was a mirror. There simply to reflect their own problems back at them. They knew absolutely nothing about me; other than the fact I can pull a banging presentation out of the bag.

Little did I know, my efforts at professional support were falling on deaf ears. Or worse, they were being actively filtered through a delusional psyche that reframed my triage into some sort of warped, consensual courtship.

I know this now, because they did it again.

This time, they decided that a static image was insufficient to convey their message. They added a whole new dimension in the form of a video file. I clicked it, assuming it might be a voice note or an apology. It was neither.

It was a performance.

They were engaged in explicit self-stimulation, staring into the lens with a terrifying intensity. The video did not cut away. It continued through to the culmination of their efforts, capturing the climax in high definition, accompanied by audio that was nothing short of grotesque.

I have to say it exactly how it was. There is no way to describe this politely, and I refuse to soften their perversion. It was an assault on the senses.

The physical rejection was instant. My body recognised the toxicity before my brain could process the visual trauma. The saliva flooded my mouth: the specific, salty warning sign that every nurse knows. I didn't just feel nauseous. I barely made it to the sink. I vomited. I offered zero response. I instituted a total communications blackout.

What followed was an agonising period of dead air. It wasn't agonising because I missed sleep. It was agonising because I was waiting for the other shoe to drop. I was in a constant state of braced anticipation, dreading the moment the phone would buzz, and the next act of the horror show would begin.

Eventually, the silence broke. The apologies finally came flooding in. But by then, the damage had metastasised.

The whole situation began dredging up unsavoury memories from my last significant breakup. It was a cocktail of toxic nostalgia. Feelings of blame, guilt, shame, remorse, and profound inadequacy started bubbling to the surface.

Rationally, I was more than capable of compartmentalising. My frontal lobe knew that these two events were infinitely separate. I knew that Mr Z was a distinct entity from my past. But my subconscious didn't get the memo. It was busily hot-wiring the emotions from the past onto the current crisis, attaching old wounds to the actions of this one, misguided individual. I couldn't shake it. It became all-consuming.

My magic rug was most definitely defunct. The mechanism had jammed, and the pile of repressed emotion was now tripping me up every time I tried to walk across the room.

Going into university continued to be a logistical nightmare. Mr Z was inconsistent when it came to attendance, which meant I never knew if I was walking into a safe zone or a minefield. I spent every journey wondering: Will he be there today? Won't he?

On arrival, I became a human radar system. I would scan every crowd walking towards me, hunting for their face so I could execute an evasive manoeuvre in advance.

The collateral damage continued. They had a core group of friends in the cohort. To stay safe, I had to disassociate myself from them. I couldn't risk the proximity. I was dreading the inevitable recommencement of our EBL sessions.

You can therefore add 'isolation' to that ever-growing list of unhelpful emotions. I was effectively quarantining myself to avoid a virus in human form.

I needed to lance the boil. The pressure was becoming critical. I cornered a good friend, a fellow student whom I trusted to hold a bucket while I purged. My intention was simply to offload. I wanted to verbally exorcise some of the emotions I was experiencing so I could get back to the business of passing the module.

Their response was a defibrillator to the system. It certainly opened my eyes.

The level of disgust they displayed was immeasurable. They sat there for a significant period, mouth open, eyes wide, paralysed by incredulity. They looked like they were witnessing a multi organ failure in slow motion.

Then came the questions. They were less questions and more horrified exclamations. "They did what?" "That's sick!" "How could they?"

After the initial shock subsided and the forensic dissection of the events began, they were adamant. I had to do something about this. They argued that this wasn't about my own sanity, although that was clearly fraying at the edges. This was a safeguarding issue. I had a duty to ensure they didn't prey on any other innocent or vulnerable women.

I listened. I consider myself to be relatively thick-skinned. I have broad shoulders and a hide like a rhino. Not much fazes me. The older I get, the less I care about how people perceive me. I have built a career and a life on the ability to absorb impact and keep moving. But my friend's reaction shone a bright, harsh light on my own ignorance. It highlighted my apparent inability to see the situation clearly. I had become so desensitised to nonsense that I had failed to register just how toxic, vile, and damaging this person's behaviour inherently was. I had normalised the abnormal.

The deliberation was complete. The peer review was in. I decided to do something about it.

The entire block had been infected by this experience. It was a low-grade fever that I failed to purge.

However, I am nothing if not stubborn. I had allotted my compulsory study time with military precision. I had submitted every assignment. I had passed all my assessments. I was now looking forward to the sanctuary of placement, twelve weeks of clinical reality, far away from the prying threat of sexual harassment and the lecture theatre.

Before I left, I decided to detonate the bomb. I decided to report them and their grievous conduct.

My first port of call was one of the EBL facilitators. They were horrified. They actively encouraged me to escalate the issue and pointed me toward the ivory tower of the Universities student administration. Duty-bound, and believing in the system, I did just that.

The response was a masterclass in gaslighting.

I suggested the evidence. The texts. The video. The unsolicited, graphic nature of it all. The administrator looked at me, sighed, and delivered a line that nearly made my brain melt. "It sounds to me like they have a soft spot for you. You should take it as a compliment."

I sat there, dumbfounded. I checked my watch to see if I had accidentally travelled back to 1953. I explained, with forced patience, that this was unsolicited. It was wholly unacceptable. It was sexual harassment.

The solution offered was technical, not behavioural. "Just block them then." "If you really want to do anything further it will need to be a formal grievance in writing." Astonished, but unnerved, I tried one last tactic. I played the safeguarding card. I tried to shine a light on the grim reality of the situation. I pointed out that if this person was successful in their nursing degree, they would be placed in environments supporting vulnerable children and adults. They would have power over people who could not defend themselves.

The administrator looked me dead in the eye. "Exactly. Do you want to be responsible for ruining this person's career before it has even begun?" The silence in the room was heavy. The victim had become the perpetrator. I was being asked to carry the weight of their future on my shoulders.

My father's voice echoed in my head. "Choose your battles wisely." I looked at the administrator. I looked at the system that was protecting a predator over a protector. I realised that this was a battle I could not win without nuking my own degree in the process.

So, I shut up. I digitally blocked them. I ignored them in person. I swallowed the injustice, and I tried to move on.

I walked out of that office feeling smaller than I have ever felt in my life. It was a conversation only. Off the record. No paper trail: just a legacy of bad advice. I had been silenced. I had been told my safety mattered less than a predator's potential career.

I walked straight into the final session of the block. I sat down. The facilitator clicked the remote to reveal the title of our next mandatory assignment. The word appeared on the screen in size 72 font.

EMPOWERMENT.

You honestly couldn't write it.

I looked at the screen. I looked around the room. Then, I let out a sound that was half-cackle, half-sob. I laughed. Almost belly laughed out loud in the dead silence of the teaching hall.

The irony was suffocating. I was now required to write three thousand academic words on the importance of giving a voice to the voiceless. I had to explain how we, as nurses, must champion the rights of the vulnerable and challenge power structures. I had to do all this immediately after being told to sit down, shut up, and take an unsolicited explicit image as a compliment.

I laughed all the way home.

I wrote the essay. I quoted the theories. I explained the vital importance of speaking truth to power.

I got a high mark, of course. Fiction has always been my stronger suit.

08

How to Be a Student Nurse and

Fly Solo

Fresh from university's masterclass in gaslighting and clutching that ironic 'A' in Empowerment like a shield, I was dispatched to my next theatre of war: Community.

It was not a destination I had ever pinned on my mental mood board. The course handbook described the placement as "managing long-term conditions and promoting independence within the home environment." That is a very polite way of saying you are about to walk into the unregulated Wild West of other people's private lives. It meant wound care, pain control, and symptom management, all performed without the safety net of a call bell or a security guard. I adjusted my tunic, checked the fuel gauge on my new to me but not new car, and prepared to get stuck in.

My mentor was a defector from the acute system, having fled the wards to chase the illusory concept of a work-life balance. In the Community, shifts were a civilised eight hours, Monday to Friday, with a rotational on call for emergencies. I could see the appeal. It meant seeing daylight. It meant seeing The Boy awake. They evangelised the autonomy of the role, swearing they would never return to the micromanaged hellscape of the Hospital. Unlike previous mentors who looked at me with the enthusiasm reserved for a smear test, they possessed a pulse. It felt like a trap, but I was desperate enough to walk into it.

We started with the usual ritual: hovering, note-taking, and the promised "See One, Do One" method. They were significantly less enthusiastic about the paperwork, treating my Practice Assessment Portfolio like a live grenade, but I assumed I could scavenge the necessary signatures from the team later. It was a deceivingly steady start until they vanished on "indefinite leave" without explanation. I didn't ask why. In this job, sudden absences are rarely good news. I was immediately reassigned to Nurse Vale, a Band 7 veteran who knew every pothole in the territory and the medical history of every resident living on them. We loaded the car like we were prepping for a siege: dressings, sharps bins, and travel mugs containing lethal doses of caffeine. Then we headed to the first address.

"Keep your wits about you," they warned, killing the engine. "Follow my lead. Try not to look shocked. And, crucially, do not touch anything unless you absolutely have to."

We wrestled with a broken gate and fought through a garden reclaimed by nature, passing a "catio" that was essentially a shanty town of rotting wood housing a colony of feral cats. The ammonia stench hit us before we even reached the back door. I had never visited a property like this, but with windows weeping greasy condensation and grey bedsheets for curtains, I knew it wasn't going to be a sanitary environment. Nurse Vale banged on the glass like the riot squad. With no answer but obvious occupation she shouldered the door open. Inside, it wasn't hoarding; it was a total cessation of hygiene. Rubbish covered every surface, defying gravity to pile up the walls.

Bodies were draped over furniture like Salvador Dalí clocks. A mangy Alsatian clicked its claws on the sticky floorboards. I scanned for an exit, but the front door was boarded up, leaving the back door as our only escape from the jungle assault course. Nurse Vale ignored the chaos and shouted at a figure face-down on the sofa. He eventually woke like a malnourished bear, rubbing his face with enough vigour to cause friction burns.

"Alright love, you again?" He gestured vaguely at the ceiling. "You're gonna have to do this in the dark. Leccy's off."

"I'll do my best," Nurse Vale replied. "Mind if we clear a space?"

He grunted a "whatever." I was dispatched to find a broom, an archaeological dig in itself, and swept a perimeter around his feet. The pile I created was a mosaic of despair: cans, loose tobacco, blackened spoons, and debris I didn't want to identify. Suddenly, the instruction not to touch anything felt less like advice and more like a survival commandment. I gripped the broom tighter. I was sweeping a minefield.

Washing our hands was out of the question. The sink was a tower of filthy pots, sealed with a glaze that looked suspiciously like vomit. The rusty taps leaked water the colour of sewage, so we bathed our hands in sanitiser instead. The patient peeled back the blanket to reveal the damage. The dressings had disintegrated, and the wounds were open, weeping a purulent green exudate and crusted with a garnish of blanket fluff and dog hair. The smell was a complex bouquet of necrosis, wet dog, and rotting food from the powerless fridge.

We established a "sterile field", a generous term for a clear patch on a dirty table, and donned our PPE. Suddenly, the patient tried to stand. Nurse Vale assisted (shoved), him back into the chair.

"What is it you can't do without for ten minutes?" she barked.

Apparently, he couldn't sit without a drink or a smoke. Nurse Vale nodded at the coffee table. I found myself acting as sommelier, handing him a half-empty bottle of whiskey and a pre-rolled cigarette. While we performed strict Aseptic Non-Touch Technique on his legs, he sat there getting intoxicated. It was the perfect tableau of Community nursing.

I had never witnessed compression therapy performed with such precision or speed. Nurse Vale wanted out. I had to haul her upright; the knees of her uniform trousers stuck to the adhesive filth of the carpet before peeling away with a grim tearing sound. We shoved the waste into a bag, cleansed as well as we could and backed towards the door.

As Nurse Vale shouted the next appointment date, I heard movement in the hall. I assumed it was another occupant waking up. Then came the voice. Small. Trembling.

"Mummy."

I froze. Framed in the shadows stood a skeletal young woman, eyes wide with terror, clutching a small boy. My instinct screamed to go to them. To scoop them up. To check them.

Nurse Vale's hand clamped around my arm like a vice. "Come on. There is nothing you can do right now."

I couldn't look away. The fear in that woman's eyes pinned me to the spot.

Nurse Vale yanked me harder, dragging me towards the daylight. "Now, Victoria. NOW."

Stepping out of that house felt like surfacing from a sewer. The fresh air didn't cleanse me; it highlighted the filth. I needed a shower. I needed to scrub my skin with wire wool.

Back in the car, the silence was absolute. We sat shell-shocked, like two soldiers after a heavy barrage.

Nurse Vale broke the trance. "Come on. There is a routine for this. I'll show you." She drove a few streets to a park. "Get out." It wasn't a request. We walked to a bench by the playground and sat. We didn't speak. We didn't need to. The breeze cooled my face, carrying the sound of children playing in the distance. Normal, happy children. The contrast with the silent boy in the dark hallway weighed heavily on my chest.

After a few minutes, she stood up.

"We have done all we can. We will report it again when we get back to the office. I will show you how. But that is all we can do."

The word "again" hung in the air, heavy with futility.

We returned to the hub. Nurse Vale, exercising their rank, went to change their uniform. I, lacking such luxury, spent the rest of the day itching. I walked into the next patient's house smelling like I had just finished a double shift in a Dutch brown cafe.

Back at the hub, while the kettle boiled, Nurse Vale introduced me to the grim administrative reality of Safeguarding. The textbook definition is noble; it speaks of "protecting human rights" and ensuring a life "free from harm." But as we clicked through the patient's history, those words felt less like a promise and more like a taunt.

The sheer volume of data was hard to comprehend. The scroll bar on the screen was microscopic, a testament to years of documented decline. Every entry was a meticulous catalogue of failure: medical non-compliance, environmental hazards, and the slow, inevitable rot of a household.

And that was only the clinical notes. The incident reports were a separate volume of horror. It was a greatest hits compilation of risk: unidentified males: aggressive and intoxicated, exposure to illicit substances, and biological hazards that would make a sanitation worker weep. Apparently, the comatose bear we met today was the patient on a good day. Usually, he wasn't so compliant.

Reading it on a screen in a warm office, the danger felt abstract. But out there, it was carnal. It opened my eyes to the specific vulnerability of the Community Nurse. We weren't just clinicians; we were trespassers in volatile territories, walking into the unknown armed with nothing but a tunic, a stethoscope, and a prayer.

If the morning was a lesson in squalor, the afternoon was a study in whiplash. We arrived at a detached bungalow that screamed "new money." The double garage displayed a fleet of cars so pristine they looked edible. The garden was manicured to within an inch of its life, boasting topiary deserving of awards and blooms that would make Chelsea judges weep.

The interior was beautifully subtle. We stepped onto marble flooring that echoed with every step. The living space was open plan, filled with custom furniture upholstered in affluence. The gold ornaments bordered on "Dictator Chic," but in this setting, the opulence somehow worked.

The patient's girlfriend opened the door. She was stunning, radiating a level of sophistication that isn't taught; it is purchased. With a landslide-victory smile, she said, "You go on through; you know where he is."

She sashayed away with the poise of a catwalk model. I stood there, still itching from the fleas of the previous house, feeling like a swamp creature.

We navigated the vast expanse of the open-plan living and crossed the manicured lawn to the "outbuilding." To call it a shed would be an insult to the entire construction industry. It was a studio of obscene proportions. One wall was a shrine to technology, housing multiple flat screens and enough speakers to power a festival.

Our patient sat in the centre of a row of plush cinema seats, looking like a slothful Captain Kirk. He wore a noise-cancelling headset and barked tactical orders into a microphone, fighting a digital war *in Call of Duty* while we stood there, waiting to treat his actual battle scars.

Nurse Vale stepped into his line of fire. He killed the game, removing his headset to reveal a beaming smile that didn't match the digital sniper he was roleplaying. "Good to see you!"

We were there to redress his residual limb, a right side, below-knee amputation. Nurse Vale supervised while I attended to the wound. He had recently started the fitting process for a revolutionary state of the art prosthetic, but the galling and sweat inside the socket had chewed up the skin, leaving it angry and ulcerated.

As I prepped the dressing, he turned his charm on me. "Ever seen a one-legged man this close up and personal?"

"Perhaps not this close," I replied, keeping my eyes on the wound to hide my awkwardness.

He lowered his voice to a sombre whisper, his face falling into a mask of tragedy. "I lost it in an accident. I was a paratrooper."

I froze. I looked at him, feeling a surge of solemnity, and delivered the most American line possible.

"Thank you for your service."
He burst into hysterics. Nurse Vale joined in, cackling as they handed me the tape.

"Nah, love!" he gasped, wiping a tear. "I got diabetes and didn't manage it but I like that story better."

"Right, let's do this," he announced. "You don't mind if I refuel?"

With a weary nod from Nurse Vale, he leaned down to a built-in cooler, because of course his modular sofa had a fridge, and retrieved the diabetic starter pack. A can of Monster and a selection of chocolate bars.

I continued the dressing, trying to ignore the irony of applying antimicrobial silver to a wound while he actively pumped sugar into his bloodstream. The wound was clinically infected, necessitating a prescription for antibiotics and a mountain of paperwork.

"Okay," Nurse Vale sighed, opening the file. "It would be remiss of me not to have the usual conversation."

"Fire away," he replied with a mock salute, cracking the ring pull on the can.

They ran through the Diabetes Risk Tool like a catechism. Have you been monitoring your blood glucose? Have you been out of range? Any dietary issues? He fired back the obligatory "correct" answers with the rhythm of a man who had memorised the cheat sheet.

They stopped and pointed their pen at his choice of hydration. "You know I have to point out the detrimental effects of that, right? It is essentially liquid gangrene."

"Listen," he shrugged, taking a bite. "Worst case scenario, I lose the other leg. If I can live without one, I can live without two."

He gestured grandly at the flat screens and the studio. "Besides, without the diabetes, I wouldn't have all this, would I?"

It transpired that the bungalow, the cars, and the cinema room were funded by a substantial clinical negligence payout for the initial missed diagnosis. He had effectively traded his lower right leg for a life of luxury and seemed perfectly willing to negotiate a price for the left one.

The next shift marked the return of my mentor, fresh from a break overseas. I was relieved to see them. I thought we had built a solid foundation, a bond that might survive the placement. I looked forward to showing off the skills I had acquired in the trenches with Nurse Vale.

However, within two visits, the atmosphere had shifted. It wasn't a step back; it was a factory reset.

It was as if we were on Day One. My role was downgraded from participant to spectator. She blocked me from patients, reverting to a strict "watch and learn" policy that left me standing in the corner, feeling more than redundant.

I chalked it up to post-holiday blues and waited. By the second day, the silence in the car was thick enough to chew. I have a decent poker face, but the tension was leaking out.

Finally, she asked, "Is there something wrong?"

I took the opening. I explained that in their absence, I had been completing treatments and gathering evidence for my portfolio. I was trying to advocate for my education.
They looked at me with annoyance. "You need to walk before you can run, Victoria. Until I see you are capable, you observe."

It was a gut punch. I was thrown back to the helplessness of my first placement. I sat there wondering what on earth I was doing wrong. The common denominator, it appeared, was me.

The rest of the day was an endurance test. Communication didn't just break down; it evaporated. I repeatedly petitioned for menial tasks, asking if I could prep dressings, unpack the boot, or act as a glorified sherpa. I was desperate to prove I wasn't dead weight to the team. The response was either a sharp "no" or total cessation of speech.

I was at a complete loss. Terrified of making the situation worse, I took a vow of silence, shrinking into the passenger seat. I spent the drive home trying to solve a puzzle with missing pieces. What had gone so spectacularly wrong?

Unable to process the lack of logic, I decided to deploy my standard coping mechanism. I lifted the corner of my mental rug, swept my feelings firmly underneath it, and tried to feign relaxation, utterly dreading whatever fresh hell tomorrow would bring.

I arrived the next morning armed with fragile optimism, only to find the portcullis still firmly down. My mentor had arrived early, reviewed the patient list, and packed the car themselves. This dismantling of our routine felt deliberate. Before their "holiday," we had a symbiotic system where I played logistics manager, allowing them to tackle the administrative mountain without working outside their scheduled hours. It was a rare win-win.

It is a universal truth that no nurse, in any setting, can complete their assigned tasks within the time allocated. The workload is a gas; it uses diffusion to fill every available second, then permeates the membrane of your personal life. You either donate your free time to the NHS, or you hand over a catastrophe to the next shift. Our previous arrangement was a survival strategy, and they had cancelled it.

Before the shift, I phoned my dad for a tactical briefing. He dispensed his standard advice, usually reserved for when I was about to do something reckless. "Do what is asked." "Keep your head down." "Do not antagonise." With that mantra in mind, I knew the real challenge of the day wouldn't be the clinical work; it would be keeping my mouth shut.

What followed was sheer agony. The pre-visit ritual of discussing patients, learning outcomes, or general life gossip was abolished. We travelled in a silence so heavy it felt structural.

I was flying blind. Arriving at each address, I had no idea if we were walking into a wound dressing or a palliative crisis. I was forced to stand like a mannequin in the corner, watching her perform every task independently. I wasn't even permitted to act as a pack mule for the equipment bags. I stood on the periphery, feeling about as useful as a chocolate fire-guard, rendered obsolete in my own education.

Whether it is a character flaw or a factory setting, my capacity for silence has a strict expiration date. I rarely raise my voice, but I possess a face that betrays my internal monologue with high-definition clarity. I pride myself on being diplomatic, yet I find that "articulate" is often mistranslated as "belligerent" by people who simply dislike the content of the message. They hear arrogance; I hear a necessary attempt to clear the air.

It wasn't the silence that was debilitating; it was the sheer weight of the atmosphere. The air in the car was thick with unsaid grievances. I found myself second-guessing every movement, paralyzed by the anxiety of not knowing which version of my mentor would respond if I dared to speak.

Without open dialogue, resolution is impossible. You can doubtless predict the trajectory of this shift. My father's advice to keep my head down was sound, but ultimately non-viable. The strategic silence flatlined. I opened my mouth and spilled the diagnosis.

I spent my hours of enforced redundancy formulating a strategy to breach the tension. I drafted scripts in my head, weighing the pros and cons of every sentence. I decided to hold fire until the last patient had been seen. It was a tactical choice. If the conversation went nuclear, I did not want to be trapped in a confined space with the fallout for the rest of the afternoon.

I prepared myself for a difficult discussion. Instead, I stepped on a landmine. And escalate, it certainly did.

We returned to the hub. They busied themselves with the patient notes while I sat watching, performing my new role as the captive audience. Once the final entry was saved, I plucked up the courage to speak.

"Could we have a quick chat?"

She checked the clock. "I have to get home. Can it wait?" She saw the obvious distress on my face and sighed with performative patience. "Go on then. But quickly."

My carefully rehearsed opening statement evaporated. Faced with their palpable reluctance, my arguments failed me. I reverted to the raw question that was bothering me. "Have I done something wrong?"

"No." The answer was flat, offered without a millimetre of elaboration.

I tried to push through. I stumbled over my words, explaining that the dynamic felt different, that I felt excluded from patient care, and asking if there was anything I could do to rectify the situation.

Their cheeks flushed with sudden anger. They snapped the words out. "Not everything is about you, Victoria. Go home. Take tomorrow as a study day. I will see you on Monday."

With that, they grabbed their bag and walked out.

I sat alone in the silence of the empty hub, feeling shell-shocked. I let the frustrated tears fall, wondering why I seemed to possess a supernatural ability to find conflict, even when I was trying my hardest not to instigate it.

The weekend was a two-day spiral of overthinking. I spent forty-eight hours wrestling with the urge to throw in the towel and walk away from nursing, absolute. Eventually, I managed to hoist up my metaphorical big girl pants and report for duty.

My mentor was not there. In fact, they weren't going to be there at all.

I was greeted by Nurse Vale. They offered a warm welcome, but it came with a chaser of dread. "Hang around here this morning, Victoria. You can work on your assignment. Someone will be in to see you shortly."

Shit, shit, shit.

The suggestion that I could productively work on an assignment was laughable. I stared blankly at the screen for what felt like an eternity, unable to focus on anything other than the gnawing anxiety of the unknown.

Hours later, the Modern Matron finally entered the hub. The title alone commands a certain level of fear. They summoned me to their office. I had only met them a handful of times, so I had no baseline to read their expression. I didn't know if this was a rescue mission or an execution, but my gut was betting heavily on the latter.

We entered the office and I stopped dead. Sitting next to the academic liaison was my academic liaison from the university.

My stomach dropped through the floor. If I could have bolted. I would have run and then when I had gotten far enough, run some more. But escape wasn't an option.

The pleasantries were brief. The Modern Matron explained that a "concern" had been raised regarding my communication skills. They emphasised the word carefully, distinguishing it from a "complaint," as if that semantic difference would lower my heart rate. The irony of being accused of poor communication by a mentor who had subjected me to a week of professional excommunication was almost impressive.

I was asked to elaborate. I decided to cling to the facts. I relayed the events of the previous week with absolute transparency, detailing the silence and the exclusion. They listened, scribbling notes like court stenographers.

When I finished, barely keeping the frustration tears at bay, the Modern Matron spoke. "Take a break. Get a coffee. Clear your head. We will call you back."

Clear my head? As if.

Summoned once more, I returned to the office. My academic liaison turned to me immediately. "Victoria, the only reason I am here is in a support role."
I felt the colour drain from my face. My heart rate pounded against my ribs. Was this it? Had I finally self-sabotaged my only hope of becoming a nurse? The internal panic was deafening. I struggled to hear them over the catastrophic screams in my head, catching only fragments of sentences, until one phrase cut through the static.

"I have no issues with your practice or communication skills. I will leave it to the Modern Matron to continue this conversation."

With that, they gathered their things and disappeared.

The Executive Matron turned to me, their voice soft and reassuring. "Okay. Now, let's take a breath."

I needed several.

They explained that in my absence, they had met with both my mentor and Nurse Vale to discuss my progress at length. It transpired that Nurse Vale was my absolute saviour. They had gone through my entire portfolio, page by page, and provided a written evidential statement. She had validated my clinical practice, patient interaction, and documentation. She didn't just defend me; she dismantled the accusations, holding my work in high regard and even offering a list of recommendations to assist my future progression.

The relief was dizzying, but the confusion remained. When asked how I felt, I admitted the events of the last week had rattled me. Despite the positive feedback from Nurse Vale, I needed to know if there was a preventative measure I had missed. Was there something I could have done differently to avoid this relationship derailment?

The Modern Matron offered a diplomatic non-answer. "All I will say is that your mentor has had some personal challenges they are working through. Their behaviour was due to preoccupation, and they are being supported."

It was standard HR code for "it's not you; it's them."

I was excused. I stood, desperate to escape before the mood changed, but they stopped me. "Hold on a minute."

I paused. They leaned forward, dropping their voice. "For the record, Victoria, but very much off the record. Be aware that exceptional students, not that I'm saying you are, can often unknowingly highlight the stagnation of others. It can lead to... certain insecurities. Do not take it all to heart."

The subtext was loud and clear. My competence was the threat. I smiled and left the office with my confidence reassembled, grateful for the reprieve and the second chance.

After the dopamine crash of the meeting, Nurse Vale sent me home early with a cryptic instruction to "prepare for tomorrow." Grateful for the escape, I went home and collapsed, ignoring the warning.

The next morning, I entered the hub to find the Modern Matron and Nurse Vale waiting. Despite the exoneration, my stomach tightened into a familiar knot. What had I done now?

Nurse Vale beckoned me to a table covered in paperwork. "Right then. Here is your patient list."

They tapped a schedule. "I have selected three for you to ease you in. All patients you have seen, assisted, and documented before. I have routed them in postcode order. Go to the furthest point and work your way back. I stocked your kit today, but from tomorrow, that is your responsibility."
I stood there, stunned by the sudden autonomy. The Modern Matron stepped forward. "This is your Lone Working Policy. Read it and sign it. And this is your Service Vehicle Use Agreement. Sign it to authorise your mileage. See you when you get back."

Without another word, she vanished.

I turned to Nurse Vale, who was standing proud. They handed me one final document. A Mentor Reassignment Agreement.

"Sign it," they smiled. "But only if you want to, that is?"

I couldn't get the pen out fast enough. It was official. I had a new mentor and a new status. I was flying solo.

For the remainder of my time in Community, the patients were mine. All mine. Naturally, Nurse Vale remained the safety net. They countersigned every action and received a comprehensive handover at the end of each day, but the operational reality was autonomy.

I finally felt like a fully-fledged nurse rather than a spare part. The surge in confidence was second to none. That validation didn't only restore my passion; it hardened my determination. It proved that I could keep going, even when the wind was blowing hard against me.

The final week marked the return of my original mentor. They greeted me with sheepish shyness, gathered their notes, and vanished. We spent the remainder of the week operating as passing ships, passively agreeing to avoid meaningful interaction.

Nurse Vale handled my paperwork. The university had finally capitulated to complaints regarding the subjective grading scale. The old system, where mentors capped scores fearing moderation, was scrapped for a binary Pass or Fail. I passed.
It was another placement with a rocky middle but a successful end. On my last day, I scraped together enough cash for a card and enough doughnuts to induce a collective sugar coma. Nurses adhere to a strict biological imperative: if cake is available, it must be eaten until it ceases to exist. It remains the gold standard of farewell gifts.

As the gathering wound down, my original mentor asked for a quick chat. I agreed, desperate to leave on good terms.

We stepped into a clinic room, but before they could speak, tears began streaming down her cheeks. They started to discuss their personal circumstances, but I gently stopped them. I reassured them that their private life was just that.

They shook their head. "It's not that, Victoria. I have failed you. You are my first student, and I didn't expect... well, you."

I wasn't sure how to take that. They clarified, "Anyone would think you were a nurse already. I didn't know how to teach you."

I told them they had been integral to my learning. I added, with absolute sincerity, that if I could become half the nurse she was, I would be proud. We hugged and vowed to stay in touch. To this day, we remain friends.

I reflected on what I loved about the placement. It was the holistic nature of the work; not just treating the patient but supporting their families through health coaching. I thrived on the autonomy and the privilege of advocating for patients to remain independent in their own homes.

What did I hate? Getting stuck in traffic. If gridlock was the only true downside, perhaps Community nursing was an option after all.

09

How to Be a Student Nurse and

Master the Art of the Pass

Flying solo had me energised. There was a discernible power in having that bit of autonomy, even if it was still shrouded in a support system. I was heading into the next university term feeling poised for once. The previous placement had done the impossible; the trust and responsibility my senior mix had awarded me with had built a newfound confidence I hadn't expected to find. I finally stopped the internal monologue of "Can I?" and started manifesting "I can" and "I am." It was a rare, moment of feeling like I might just belong in a clinical setting.

That was, until I was introduced to the world of OSCEs. In nursing, this acronym is treated with the same superstitious dread as the word "quiet" on a night shift. You know it is relevant, non-negotiable, and vital. It is one of the grim pinnacles of nurse training; without a definitive pass, you simply are not a nurse. But mentioning it or discussing it out loud triggers a specific brand of fear. It takes the usual mix of student anxiety and clinical nausea to a level that feels like you're staring down the barrel of a life sentence for a crime you haven't committed yet.

I even bought a book. I would refer to it now to help remind myself of the sheer horror of studying for this exam, but I can't. I gifted it to a student nurse I discovered sobbing in the staff room the day before their assessment. They looked the way I felt, like they were mourning their own future. I could have bought another copy for future reference, but if I hadn't given it away, I probably would have burnt it in some sort of freedom ritual. There are some objects that carry too much of a scent of failure to keep in your house.

Objective. Structured. Clinical. Examinations. These four words would haunt you for the entirety of your career. Even though you would eventually drag yourself through this pass or fail assessment, you would revisit the scene many times in your head. Sometimes you imagined yourself performing with the rhythmic, mechanical precision of a human metronome on a chest cavity, and other times with the panicked, useless clumsiness of someone trying to catheterise a horse.

This was the very core of how to deal with a life and death situation. It was the one and only time you were expected to demonstrate every single skill university had drilled into you, all at once. You were juggling clinical technique, communication, professionalism, data interpretation, management, and the kind of high-stakes maths that usually requires a quiet room and three double espressos. You had to do it all while being watched, trying your absolute hardest not to kill a plastic mannequin, throw up, or have a catastrophic faecal accident.

Add to this a large, open-plan gymnasium sectioned off into stations, each one highly visible to everyone else. It was designed so that anyone with a vested interest in seeing you fail could sit court side and watch the collapse in real time, perhaps taking some small comfort in the knowledge that they were not alone in their incompetence.

A crowd-strong line of delegates waited in a grim queue, everyone fidgeting with the same wired energy while awaiting their fate. Standing at the stations were some of the most knowledgeable clinical educators you would ever face, pens poised over clipboards like judges at a particularly morbid talent show. It was a very real, very drafty version of hell on earth.

Waiting in line presented you with a limited selection of options for the patience game. You could try to stand quietly and breathe deeply, attempting to think of anything other than the stack of post-it notes you had dotted at every eye-level surface in your house.

Those neon squares of paper haunted your life: stuck above the kettle while you waited for it to boil, plastered to the fridge door when you were trying to talk yourself out of binge eating or downing a bottle of wine, and taped to the bathroom mirror where you stared at them while too exhausted to dry yourself after a cold shower. They were the wallpaper to your mid-life evaluation.

That method of silent zen would be perfectly plausible if it wasn't for the fact that you were surrounded by every other quivering wreck in the cohort. Their panic was infectious, a low-frequency hum of impending doom that made your own preparation feel like a house of cards in a tornado.

The next option was to talk. Incessantly. You babbled about nothing of any importance. It was meaningless drivel intended to let you zone out. It provided enough energy to feign engagement without letting your brain pivot back to the clinical points you'd convinced yourself you'd forgotten. It was a necessary distraction to prevent a total nervous system implosion. It required zero intellect and even less of a meaningful thought process. You weren't conversing. You were filling the silence, so the panic didn't have room to breathe.

Alternatively, you could try blind panic. You could ask everyone to start reciting their study methods to you, but I warn you that this would only end in one student mentioning a part of the process you had never heard of. This discovery would render you mentally incapable of speaking, let alone saving lives. Don't do this one. It was a one-way ticket to catatonia before you'd even picked up a blood pressure cuff.

You could choose my option. I started counting the number of people in the line ahead of me. With a definitive number of stations required to pass, I put my maths to the test. I worked out an average time for each assessment, divided it by the number of people before me, and calculated an expected time of arrival. I correlated this with the actual time and prayed that I was at least the penultimate student before the break.

My theory was that the assessors would be so bored of the repetition that their thirst and hunger triggers would take over. I hoped they might start passing people without the same vigour they had when they were bright-eyed, bushy-tailed, fed and hydrated. It didn't really help with anything other than practising for the medication calculation round, but it kept my mind occupied.

And then there you were. Next up. The first assessor peered at you. You stood there. They peered some more. You waited until they shouted "next" with the same vigour you were supposed to use when shouting for help at the first station.

Basic Life Support. It was the very core of life-saving protocol, yet you still managed to confuse "Stayin' Alive" with "Nellie the Elephant." I always found I sang one faster than the other. It meant I was either going to save your life or give you a pointless chest massage during your last breaths.

You instinctively forgot right from left. Is it my left or the patient's, right? Where is the heart? You second-guessed everything. Adults and children, rescue breaths or not, and if so, how many? Is this the latest updated protocol? By the time you'd forced your brain into some semblance of order, you realised you'd forgotten to call for help or check for hazards. Every second felt like an eternity. While you were busy contemplating your next move, your mannequin had potentially expired.

You emerged a hot, sweaty mess and were immediately expected to accurately interpret a drug chart scrawled by a doctor in a state of terminal, sleep-deprived velocity. You had to select the correct medication and dispense the tablet without touching it or pinging it across the room in blind panic. Then, you had to explain the purpose of the drug, its common side effects, and the administration protocol.

Whatever you do, don't drop the pill. If it hit the floor, you were sucked into the inquisitorial vortex of re-administration, medication counts, missing medication disposal, and endless documentation. One slip of the finger and you'd traded clinical care for an afternoon of paperwork and shame.

The next goal was to structure a comprehensive, holistic, and safe care plan. You had to write the whole thing out without dropping your biro or sweating all over your freshly penned ink. You were desperately trying to maintain a level of legibility that suggested a professional clinician rather than a primary school student having a tantrum with a crayon. It was difficult to focus when you were all-consumed by whether you remembered to sign the box for the PRN paracetamol at the last station, or whether you broke the ribs of your first patient because you got into excitable disco mode and defaulted to "Stayin' Alive."

It was all fine, though. In the real world, if someone is in cardiac arrest, your BLS training kicks in like I imagine a line of cocaine would before the beat drops. Medication administration becomes an ingrained, reflex setting. It is eventually easier than riding a bike, provided the bike isn't a unicycle.

As for care planning, you would have all the time in the world to complete it thoroughly at the end of your shift. Usually, this happened once you had already clocked off but were legally tethered to the building until every box was ticked.

In a macabre kind of way, the pressure of the OSCEs provided a relative relief from my current reality. I was still recovering from the aftermath of that random, unsolicited sexual gesture and the total lack of support from the people meant to protect us.

The sheer depth of study and application had served as a distraction. The anger and injustice continued to sit in the pit of my stomach and the back of my mind. It occasionally reminded me of its existence, but it was not enough to deter me from the end goal. Resilience is so embedded in the nursing world that it is documented as a cold hard fact into the Code of Conduct. If that wasn't the truest test of that requirement, I didn't know what was.

Finally, our clinical skills were beginning to get a real hammering. You would still most likely walk out of the university not knowing how to find a vein, place a cannula, or take bloods. But apparently, you could pick that up on your own on day one as a registered nurse after seeing it done once.

You would also have never placed a male urinary catheter on anything other than the rubber dildos provided in training. You could move and manipulate those any which way without causing physical pain or permanent erectile dysfunction so you would still be unequipped to do so on a human.

You might encounter a rogue mentor along the way who took pity on you and your pathetic range of skills. Knowing full well what was to come, they might illegally allow you to try such things on a living human, but that was never to be spoken about. Ever.

To support this clinical training, we were to complete a simulated anatomy and physiology session on cadavers. Actual, real people. They were dead, but very, very real. Trying to deny my excitement at this prospect would be a blatant lie. I appeared to have unwittingly segregated myself into a distinctly labelled group of weirdos by expressing joy at the thought of dissecting something other than a rat.

While others looked positively pallid, I went in with an air of buoyancy, wondering if we had to put all the bits back in.

It was epic. Odd. Surreal. It was strangely satisfying and riveting all at the same time. I knew livers were large but bugger me. The one we manhandled out of an abdominal cavity was bigger than a rugby ball and weighed about the same as both of my cats put together. It was a heavy, stark revelation of what the human body can house.

It served as a perfect, if slightly gruesome, discussion point. As we worked, we reviewed the patient's clinical history, realising they had spent years living on a diet consisting of full fat everything and alcoholic meal supplements. Seeing the physical toll of those choices laid out in front of you is a far better teacher than any textbook. And don't even get me started on the intestinal tract. Once that was out and unravelled, there was no chance of a tidy exit. That thing was definitely not going back in.

The division in the room was immediate and absolute. Some of us excelled, diving in with a morbid curiosity that probably should have been alarming. Others baulked at the mere thought of touching the greasy, preserved insides of a formaldehyde-soaked stranger, standing a few feet back with their hands tucked firmly under their armpits.

Then there were those who full on wiped out. It starts with the "cadaver sway," where a student begins to rock gently on their heels before the colour drains from their face, leaving them the same shade of grey as the person on the table. One minute they were looking at a gallbladder, and the next they were being pulled out in a drag lift to go and lie on a cold corridor floor.

With the clinicals almost all signed off, it was back to the lecture theatres for assignment prep. Once more into the breach. The brief, primal thrill of the anatomy lab was over, replaced once more by the slow, soul-crushing reality of referencing and word counts.

We were now deep into the preparation for what we thought was the final piece of work. This was the academic culmination of proof. The Literature Review. I say "thought" because we eventually discovered that this mammoth piece of soul-destroying theory comparison was merely the prequel to a Quality Improvement assignment.

I viewed the title as a last-ditch attempt to finally have my say. It was a chance to offer a suggestion or evidence-based independent thought. I was desperate for something other than a repetitive cycle of "he once said" being counteracted by "she once did."

If you overthink the Literature Review, you were doomed. You were setting yourself up for a terminal panic attack. It was one of those moments where you truly believed you were in cardiac arrest and found yourself wondering if you could perform life-saving skills on yourself.

In a perfect world, you should pre-plan. You should plan some more and then, once you have a clear structure, plan again. You need to dissect the grading criteria to see exactly what the examiners want. Break down each point, relate it to your research, and apply a strict word count to every section. You must not waffle. You must not fluff. Most importantly, do not write a single word that cannot be referenced.

Approaching it in bite-size, manageable chunks makes the work feel a world away from the overwhelming chunk of words standing between you and the professional healthcare sector. It was the difference between becoming a nurse or trotting off to work in a supermarket. This was a great plan and worked very well unless you were me. I ignored the bloody thing until a few weeks before the deadline. While I eventually followed the structure I outlined, I did so at record speed within the twilight zone of many sleepless nights.

Here was the next piece of gargantuan advice. When selecting a topic, choose one that has been done countless times before. No, scrap that. Choose one that has been exhausted to death. You will learn very quickly that the research element of this project is practically the whole thing. It is not just the research itself that matters, but the pivotal academic proof of how you conducted it. You must justify your methodology with the fervour of a Matron defending the sanctity of their ward.

You must explain which research tools you used, the demographic you selected, and the reasoning behind your every choice, even if that decision was ill-informed. Then, you have to carefully dissect this down into a handful of relevant papers that cover your subject matter to either prove or disprove your objective.

Naturally, I ignored the easy path. I chose "Antimicrobial Therapy in the Community: A Strategy to Support Admission Avoidance and Reducing Delayed Discharges." Aside from a handful of defunct trials that had already collapsed, I found it almost impossible to explain why I had narrowed my selection down to a small handful of specific papers. There were barely a few in total to choose from in the entire world. I passed, but only after my academic advisor pointed out that I really should have stuck to the benefits of routine screening for diabetes in older adults. It would have saved me a lot of grey hairs and several late-night metabolic crises.

When you had finally hit your word count, got the bloody thing handed in, and decided to never revisit the topic again, the university moved the goalposts. You were forced to dredge up every last painstaking element of that work and write yet another assignment on exactly how you would execute this brilliant, done a million times before project. In my case, I was attempting to develop an only done a handful a failed times trying to prove I had the academic kudos to revolutionise IV medication administration protocol.

The concept I had chosen had never been proven as anything other than a big fat waste of public money. It was impossible to effectively manage in a clinical setting and lacked any real unit admission data to ratify the results to. It was, for all intents and purposes, defunct before I even started.

The experience did, however, instil an odd interest in the murky world of health economics. I tucked that away in the back of my mind as a safety net. I figured that if all else fails and I get struck off in my first year for a terminal case of insubordination, I would at least have an alternative career option hidden within the spreadsheets of the NHS.

Finally, was the dreaded Safe Medicate Examination. The university powers that be seemingly left it right until the very end as a final, cruel test of tenacity for reasons that remain unbeknownst to me. With a mandatory full-mark pass rate, this digital demonstration of skill had been the sudden and unceremonious downfall of many an exceptional bedside nurse. It was the academic equivalent of a sudden-death penalty shootout where the goalposts were moving, and the ball was on fire.

The pressure was immense. If you could not titrate a medication down to a decimal point that had more zeros than a quadrillion, you may as well have spent the last few years backpacking around the world. You could have been living off tinned food and sleeping in beach huts instead of staring at a computer screen in a cold sweat. You might not come out of that particular life choice with any form of career prospects, but you would have possessed the life experience of countless student nurses put together. Better yet, you would no longer have had the need to be taught about the fundamentals of kindness via

PowerPoint. You would have seen it in the wild, rather than through a mandatory module.

"A full mark?" I hear you cry. Surely, they couldn't possibly mean that. But yes, they absolutely do. Do not underestimate the sheer, clinical coldness of this requirement. If you fail once, you were granted a second attempt. Fail twice, and you had the joy of mandatory remediation before enduring the battle once more. However, if you fail a third time, you entered a world of severe academic consequence that made a prison sentence look like a spa day.

In plain terms, failing the module meant you could not practise. You could not progress to the next year, which was largely irrelevant anyway because that was the final hurdle. The real upshot was that you were withdrawn from the course. Period. After a few years of blood, sweat, and placement-induced tears, you were simply done. Out. Finished. All those thousands of hours of work vanished because you misplaced a decimal point on a screen. Admittedly, that decimal point in the real world could cause multi-system organ failure, but hey, we were always told that humans made mistakes, right? Apparently, that rule applied to everyone except a student nurse with a calculator.

This environment had me thinking back to the dreaded waiting-in-line dilemma from the previous OSCEs. Only this time, you were all shoehorned into a computer suite with row upon row of monitors. They were all close enough to feel uncomfortable but not quite close enough to see anyone else's answers without causing a significant neck-strain injury. It was a room filled with the rhythmic, frantic clicking of mice and the heavy scent of communal desperation.

The next problem was your password. For security purposes, you had to change this an endless number of times, usually involving a convoluted mix of your first pet's middle name and the year you lost your dignity. It was not until you had had it on repeat for the last few days in an obsessive-compulsive ritual that you sat down, entered it, and the computer said "No." You felt your face redden and your eyes sting. "Clammy palms" was a polite way of saying you were shitting bricks. You started blindly adding capital letters, alphanumerics, and special characters until you hit capacity and the system locked you out with a smug, digital finality.

You had no choice but to wave your sweaty palm around for an adjudicator while every other student in the room stared at you. You could practically hear them thinking that if you couldn't even get into the computer, how the fuck were you going to pass a high-stakes exam? This was where a true test of your future nursing ability kicked in. You had to remember that there was no such thing as a stupid question, there was no shame in asking for help, and, most importantly, every human being makes mistakes. The only requisite was that it really depended on how big that mistake was and whether it involved a patient or a generic desktop.

Then the questions began. They came at you one after the other, each appearing achievable, some almost suspiciously simple. But in a nurse's mind, "simple" was a synonym for "trap." You started second-guessing yourself, over-analysing the very tasks you had successfully completed countless times on the wards. Administer 1g. Tablets come in 500mg. How many tablets? It was elemental arithmetic, yet the pressure rendered you a functional illiterate. Even the easiest computations had you counting on your fingers like a toddler and obsessively checking that you had selected the digital image of a tablet rather than a capsule. You clicked and re-clicked a dozen times before finally daring to hit submit.

Then the imposter syndrome began to rise, triggered by the frantic clattering of a keyboard nearby. Why the hell was she typing so fast? I was only clicking two buttons: the answer and submit. What on earth were people typing? Was I doing something so obviously wrong? Had I completely missed a secret section of the exam?

Whatever you do, do not attempt to look at anyone else's screen. I caught a glimpse of one out of the corner of my eye and saw a different background colour and larger boxes. Panic flared instantly. Why didn't mine look like that? Was I even in the right goddamn exam? All this served to do was render you useless. You had to be you, do you, and focus only on you. Distraction in this room was the epitome of failure.

Get done. Get out. And most importantly, forget about it. Avoid the groups that inevitably siphoned off into the corridor to compare notes. All you would be faced with was a barrage of "What did you put for question thirty-seven?" and "What dosage per hour did you get for the patient weighing under the threshold?" These are daily dose calculations you couldn't even remember completing. At this stage, ignorance was not just bliss; it was survival. My mother taught me a mantra that I had carried through life: there was no point worrying about something you could not change.

You were then expected to carry on regardless. You had to remain engaged, studying and working non-stop. You were faced with your next bout of unpaid labour on placement, all whilst wondering if that one exam was the one that would end this entire three-year journey, leaving you with nothing but the bitter taste of failure. Waiting for the online portal to buffer before your grade downloads was worse than watching a banking app prepare to tell you that you had nil pounds. Then, finally, the screen cleared. Full marks. And breathe. You were still in the game!

10

How to Be a Student Nurse and

Not Crumble in Front of the Gods

I found it difficult to describe the feeling of donning a fresh pair of scrubs. Slipping your feet into a pair of Crocs and walking the halls of theatres. You feel invincible. Heroic, even. I can't lie; it grants you a sense of total autonomy. For some, that translated into plain self-satisfaction; for others, it was unapologetic arrogance.

I always remember the theatre teams frequenting other areas of the Hospital in their pristine gowns worn back-to-front. They flaunted personalised caps they were strictly forbidden from wearing outside the OR, simply because they could. It was like watching the Red Sea part. People could not help but stare, as if some higher power had entered the room. The truth was, they had. These were the people who held life in their hands. Literally.

Apprehensive about this placement was an understatement and about as far removed from my comfort zone as a misanthrope at a mandatory staff party. I could only compare being in the presence of a consultant to having a live wire housed in my cranium: It was all consuming enthral, a cocktail of adoration and fear. The fear was logical, grounded in the fact they held as much knowledge in one brain cell as I did in my entire head. Their volume of expertise was extraordinary. When teamed with an ability to complete physical tasks with ultimate precision, I was rendered speechless through sheer reverence.

For those of you going into a theatre placement, I advise you to practise speaking to the people who intimidate you most. When a consultant finally asks you for something, the last thing you want to do is shit yourself.

I typically divide consultants into two categories: ones that teach and ones that don't. This means you have some that will speak and others that will simply bark. You must learn to adapt your communication style to accommodate them at all times. You could, if you so wish, professionally challenge them. It is an approach I usually champion, but in theatres, you do so at your own peril. Be prepared for the consequences: a student nurse challenging a senior clinician is roughly equivalent to a field mouse filing a formal complaint against a combine harvester.

Theatre nurses are an entirely different breed. If the consultants are the gods of this environment, the scrub team are the high priests who keep the temple from burning down. For your placement, there are some survival tips I can offer you: if you think you are organised, multiply your skills by one hundred. If you think your personal hygiene is perfect, scrub twice. If you think you speak clearly and concisely, reduce your sentence word count by fifty percent.

This group of nurses are specialised, highly trained, and take no prisoners. They monitor the environment with a terrifying, hawk-like intensity. They count how many minutes a surface has been disinfected with the same lethal precision they apply to counting surgical swabs. To understand their mindset, think portion control down to the exact number of peas on a plate. If one pea is missing, the entire system stops until it is found. They are the guardians of the sterile field, and if you accidentally breathe on their tray, you might as well start drafting your will.

If you so much as look at a drape in the field, you will have eyes upon you. Do not walk towards it, around it, or anywhere near it unless expressly asked to do so. Touch it and you will spontaneously combust, set on fire by the collective glare of the room.

If your nose itches, ignore it. If your glasses fall down the bridge of your nose, leave them there. If you have something in your eye, blink it out. The second you touch your face, prepare to de-robe and scrub in all over. If they even let you, that is.

I was on a Urology rotation. As you might expect, that involved everything to do with the lower urinary system: a world of bladders, kidneys, and things I would explain in more detail later. For now, we focused on day one. After an induction and a brief introduction to my mentor two shifts prior, I was prepared for a day of shadowing routine surgeries. Or so I thought.

The Theatre Manager gathered all the student nurses at the central hub. We stood there and waited. Then we waited some more. We looked like a collection of rabbits caught in headlights, all far too terrified to speak. Finally, they explained that a radical microvascular reconstruction was being performed by one of the countries leading consultants. They had authorised two students to observe.

"Since it is day one and I don't know any of you yet," they said, "I'll have to settle this by a show of hands and random selection."

I didn't have the foggiest clue what a microvascular reconstruction was. However, before they could even finish the sentence, my hand was firmly in the air. I used every mm of my 5ft 11" to my advantage. I was in. The operation was due to commence in two hours and was expected to last most of the day. Prep time meant research, food, and drink. Strictly in that order.

My advice for this stage is simple: research the generalised version of the procedure. Do not bog yourself down in the granular intricacies of the surgery or you will drive yourself mad. Instead, look at when it was developed and by whom. Briefly check how the methods have advanced to the current standard.

If you know the name of your surgeon: google them immediately. All medical professionals have an ego, and consultants are no exception. They are invariably gratified if you can drop a strategic line like: "I found your paper on such-and-such and used it as a reference point in an assignment."

This exact tactic once landed me the opportunity to observe the Senior Urology Consultant lead a teaching session on technology-assisted surgery. It was revolutionary, and it only cost me ten minutes of light stalking on a journal database.

You must eat, even if you aren't hungry. Once you cross the threshold into theatre, there is no going back. Most of the day is a long time, and it feels significantly longer if your stomach is rumbling. I once went into a surgery expecting a two-hour stint, but complications hit and we were trapped for six.

The embarrassment of my digestive system sounding like an artic lorry driving past at high speed could have been entirely avoided. Go for rich foods for longevity. Prioritise proteins, fibre, and healthy fats. Despite the fact you won't move for what feels like an eternity, your brain and your blood sugar are going to need the energy. Standing still is, paradoxically, exhausting.

I don't need to tell you this because you already know, but I will say it anyway: stay hydrated. I am mainly reiterating this because nurses are our own worst enemies. We are the masters of "do as we say, not as we do."

Note that staff rotate breaks, and if you aren't currently in the sterile field, you don't have to re-scrub. However, if a fast track arises to assist within that field and you aren't already scrubbed, you won't be the one selected to support the team. I once lost out on a mammoth opportunity because I vanished for four minutes to get a drink. That went into my journal as a permanent note to self: pick your moments wisely. In theatres, being in the right place at the right time is usually the difference between watching the ceremony and touching it.

***

A high-risk tissue removal involves the removal of target tissue from the chest. It is a protective measure for people who carry or are at high risk of carrying mutated risk genes. In this specific case, the patient had already faced the full litany: a malignant diagnosis, chemotherapy, radiotherapy, and the removal of lymph nodes. They were in remission, but to kill off any chance of recurrence, they had opted for a double mastectomy combined with a microvascular reconstruction.

The reconstruction is essentially a procedural heist. It involves harvesting soft tissue from the abdomen to rebuild the chest. Invented by a senior innovator in the early two-thousands, it is a microsurgical feat that requires the kind of skill usually reserved for watchmakers or bomb disposal experts.

Because all soft tissue needs a blood supply to stay alive, the consultants focus on the feeder vessels, specifically the deep lower abdominal artery and the superficial lower abdominal vein. These vessels pierce the core muscle to supply the skin and the subcutaneous layer. During the reconstruction, they are reconnected to corresponding vessels at the recipient site.

Since each muscle has its own supply and one side is often stronger than the other, the team doesn't guess blindly. The patient underwent a flow ultrasound before the first incision was even made. The most viable abdominal vessels were located, documented, and the patient's skin was marked. It was a biological map, ensuring the consultants knew exactly where to dig before the clock started ticking.

Everything was set. The team were already scrubbed in, and the draped operating tables were laden with an artillery of tools and contraptions that looked like a sadomasochist's wet dream. The room smelled of aggressive chemical cleanliness under lights so bright they felt like a physical weight.

Gowned and masked, we stood with our hands crossed over our chests. I scanned the room, taking in a sea of clean uniformity that felt uncomfortably like a scene from *The Handmaid's Tale*. The ritual of the scrub had already stripped us of our individuality. The repeated, rhythmic abrasion of the brush across my skin and the scalding water had been a transition. It was the moment I shed Victoria the student and became a silent, clean component of the suite artillery. Underneath the layers of polypropylene and latex, I could feel my own heartbeat. It was the only thing in the room that felt organic.

After what felt like an eternity, the anaesthesiologist popped their head around the door to check our status. The lead scrub nurse signalled we were ready. The double doors swung wide, and the patient was wheeled in from the prep room. They looked like a small, still figure amidst a forest of chrome and plastic. The surgical lead ran through a series of checks. A muffled drone of monitors and the hiss of the ventilator became the soundtrack. We were ready. Then we waited.

The silence was deafening. I began to feel a creeping sense of nervousness, though I couldn't quite pin down why. Being this up close and personal in such an environment is a volatile mix of excitement and overwhelm. It is underscored by a very real sense of imposter syndrome. I felt like a child wearing their parent's oversized clothes, waiting for someone to notice I didn't belong. While the team meticulously documented their instrument checks, the main event began.

Two consultants appeared from the utility room. They stood at the entrance like statues of the gods while they were gowned and gloved by the team. Their movements were minimal and efficient. It was slightly less dramatic than an episode of *Grey's Anatomy*, but damn near close. They approached the huddle with the confidence and purpose of a celebrity on a red carpet.

The lead scrub nurse announced the patient details, identified the planned procedure, and completed the final checks. Everyone nodded in agreement. When the nurse asked if there were any contentions, I felt the same spike of nerves you get when a minister asks if anyone knows why a bride and groom should not be wed. I half-expected someone to burst in with a proclamation of clinical adultery. But silence prevailed. Since this removal and reconstruction was bilateral, at least we didn't have to double-check our lefts and rights to ensure we weren't about to cut the wrong tit off. It was time.

So it began. This specific procedure requires two consultants working in perfect conjunction. The lead consultant performs the double-sided tissue removal while the second consultant, who is by no means an assistant, begins the delicate harvest of the microvascular tissue transfer from the abdomen.

I don't know if what I am about to say should matter in a clinical sense. To some, perhaps it shouldn't, but it mattered immensely to me: both lead clinicians were women. They weren't only leaders in their field; they were fierce trailblazers, commanding the room with a quiet, absolute authority.

I never thought I would hear the words spoken out loud, but when they came, they sounded as if the volume had been turned to maximum. "Ten blade." The request resonated around the clean room with an echo as magnified as if we were standing in the Grand Canyon.

As the scalpel touched the exposed flesh of the patient, the next command followed immediately: "Start clock."

Whether you've watched every medical TV drama and documentary going, or spent hours discussing clinical theory with fellow students, no one can truly predict their reaction to a sight they've never seen until it is happening six inches from their face. I've never been the type to shy away from blood or guts, but this was on another level of visceral reality.

My fellow student began to look panicked. They looked away, beads of sweat forming on their brow under the harsh suite lights. I leaned in and whispered, "Just breathe." They stared at me, desperate for encouragement. "It will pass," I promised. They thanked me using only their eyes.

Little did I know that the roles would be reversed very, very soon. Nothing. And I mean absolutely nothing, could prepare your senses for the smell of burning flesh as the diathermy began its work.

Cautery is a procedural technique that uses high-frequency electrical currents to cut or coagulate tissue. It is also responsible for yet another indescribable odour the human body is capable of producing. I will give it a bash: think of an electrical fire combined with an ulcerated wound and a generous helping of spoiled red meat. It is totally immersive, though you do eventually get used to it.

Now the real work commenced. It was time to buckle up. This was a once-in-a-lifetime opportunity: transfixing, thrilling, and god-damn show-stopping. But standing for most of the day when you were fundamentally not doing anything felt like running a physical endurance test without taking a single step.

Usually, my primary concern was my concentration span. I was worried I would get bored, disengaged, or start doing that thing where you try to hide a yawn. You know the ones: you fight it so hard to stifle it that your eyes well up with tears and they stream uncontrollably down your face. Only problem is, in this instance you are absolutely forbidden from wiping them away.

As it turned out, my attention span was the least of my problems. All thoughts gradually turned to my popliteal fossa slowly inversing, lumbago setting in, and what felt like glowing embers in the balls of my feet. I was certain those embers would be a blazing forest fire by hour three.

Four hours down and halfway through. The double-sided tissue removal was complete and the abdominal tissue for the microvascular tissue transfer had been harvested. Now for the magic. If I hadn't seen this with my own eyes, I was not sure I would have believed it was possible. The crude version was that these consultants literally created a tits out of a tummy.

I couldn't help but stand there and wonder. It felt as if a cacophony of questions had been unleashed in my brain, making logical thought an impossibility. How would they restore the blood flow? How did you stop that flow in the first place, and for how long? How did they divide the tissue so that each side was of equal size and shaped evenly? What if they hadn't harvested enough tissue to go around?

The list went on and on. I haven't written this book to provide a scientific manual or a step-by-step procedural guide, so all I will say is that every one of my questions was answered with clinical precision. I urge you to research this microscopic choreography. If you ever get the chance to witness it, jump at it. It is the closest thing to a miracle you will ever see performed with a needle and thread.

Once the consultants had finished their meticulous embroidery and the final sutures were tied, the atmosphere in the room shifted from high-tension focus to a quiet, fatigued awe. The patient was no longer a series of anatomical puzzles to be solved. They were a person who was about to wake up to a brand-new reality.

In the recovery bay, the magic of the microvascular reconstruction met the cold, hard reality of nursing care. This was not a standard post-op check. We were not only looking for a pulse; we were looking for the survival of the harvest. We monitored those new reconstructions with the intensity of a hawk watching its nest. Every hour, we checked the flap for warmth, colour, and capillary refill. If that tissue turned dusky or cold, it meant the microsurgical heist had failed. It meant the blood was not flowing.

There was a profound psychological weight to this specific recovery. The patient went under the knife to lose a part of themselves that had become a threat. They woke up with a reconstruction that used their own soft tissue to restore what the malignancy tried to steal. It was a strange, beautiful irony. The softness of their abdomen, something most of us complain about in the mirror, became the very thing that made them feel whole again.

Watching that first moment of realisation, when a patient finally feels the weight and warmth of the reconstruction, was a career highlight. It was a reminder that while the consultants played with technology and controls, the real victory happened in the quiet hours of the night. It was in the recovery room where the clinical success became a personal enlightenment.

***

Another day and another busy morning of back-to-back routine procedures was drawing to a close. I was sitting in the suite mess, inhaling my lunch, when my mentor approached and asked if they could join me. After a few minutes of general chit-chat, they asked if I would like to observe an uncommon, non-routine surgery that afternoon.

As if I was going to turn that down.

I eagerly asked for the details. My mentor looked at me, took their glasses off, and raised a single eyebrow. They had what I could only describe as a smirk: a cheeky, crooked smile with a very knowing look. Their parting words were, "Go in with an open mind and learn lots." It was as if they were desperately trying not to laugh out loud while maintaining a shred of professional decorum.

We were all professionals. However, there was no denying that a healthy level of gallows humour was necessary to get most of us through a highly pressured shift. Know that this form of benign violation never relates to a patient from a personal perspective. Also, know that there is a time and a place. And apparently, that place was whichever theatre I was heading into next.

I headed down and joined the team in the suite. I offered to assist, but since I hadn't worked with this specific crew before, they simply advised me to get scrubbed and ready. While I was at the sink, I kept hearing the term "BXO" thrown around. This was yet another procedure I had no clue about and absolutely no time to research. I couldn't shake the feeling that my mentor had omitted the details for a very specific reason. That reason was about to be revealed.

With the team ready, the patient was wheeled in from the prep room. The team kicked into gear, draping the patient and performing the rhythmic count of the instruments. Once the checks were complete, the consultant approached the table. With the help of the second clinician, they began assembling a contraption that looked like an industrial metal single-hole punch. I stood there thinking: What on fuck is that?

In time, I learned that the shorthand stands for Balantis Xerotica Obliterans, and the bizarre instrument was a compression clamp. At the time, I was still none the wiser. I moved over to the theatre circulator who was frantically punching data into the computer and quietly asked what the surgical intervention involved. They replied in a thick Aussie accent.

"Imagine a sausage that has been left on the barbie for too long," they whispered. "Like, I mean, waaaaay too long. Well, we're going to take the burnt bits off."

I was rarely speechless. In that moment, I was.

The compression clamp was a piece of procedural engineering that looked like it belonged in a nineteenth-century workshop rather than a modern operating room. It consisted of a base plate, a rocking stirrup, and a heavy tightening nut. The consultant assembled this machine around said anatomy. Watching them use it was like watching a master craftsman at a lathe.

As much as I would love to walk you through the mechanics of the Gomco clamp, I fear that might be a step too far even for my stomach. If you wish to indulge yourself, You Tube is an excellent resource. Tip; don't eat first. All you need to know is that this incredible piece of engineering enabled the consultant to essentially evacuate the organ from the pelvis, elongate it, and hold it in position. It was a brutal necessity. Because the fibrosing disease had turned the skin into something resembling calcified leather, the consultant needed the tissue to be perfectly taut and bloodless before they could begin the delicate task of debridement.

The clamp exerted a massive amount of pressure to crush the tissue at the incision site, which served two purposes. It marked the line of travel for the consultant and provided a bloodless field. Seeing a human organ being manipulated with such mechanical force was jaw-dropping. It looked like a biological heist.

Then came the "removing of the burnt bits" part. This was achieved using the consultant's answer to virtually every complication: the diathermy. For you to gain some form of mental picture, think of it as being hung like a kebab and stripped like peeling the skin from a cucumber with a hot iron poker.

At this stage, I had a vague idea of what was occurring but no real understanding of the logistics. To remedy this, I positioned myself at the foot of the bed for a front-row seat. In hindsight, having seen this done once, I would suggest a more distant vantage point should the chance ever arise. Though, statistically, it was highly unlikely: this diagnosis only affected a fraction of the population.

"Eye-watering" was the only term that fit. I didn't even possess the organ in question, yet I felt a phantom sympathetic pain as the consultant began the prep. Broadly speaking, the condition was a chronic inflammatory disease that primarily affected the outer tissue and tip of the most primary and sensitive organ most men formulate their decision making processes in.

By the time they were finished, the transformation was incredible. It was a total restoration of function hidden behind a terrifyingly raw violent exposure.

During the post-op debrief, the consultant explained that this was the most severe case they had ever witnessed. There was an abnormal growth of scarred tissue, raised, thickened skin, encasing the tip and outer tissue. It had also spread to the deep erectile tissue. The shaft was so heavily involved that the urethra was almost entirely obstructed. Due to the understandable embarrassment of the patient, they had presented late. This was the only way to ensure he would ever piss without a catheter or spunk without a purpose, ever again.

This was where things got a little bit hairy. Remember when I mentioned there was a time and a place? While we were in the thick of it, another consultant knocked on the door and walked in. They were suited and booted, holding a mask over their face, and clearly needed to consult with the operating surgeon.

As they moved as close to the clean field as possible without the leas scrub nurse hemi spherically imploding, a look of sheer surprise took over their features. "Good god, how did you get that out?" they asked. "That is the worst case I have ever seen." They were smirking audibly as they said it. I suppose they felt that laughing out loud would have been inappropriate.

I looked around the room and saw a sea of wide eyes. Arms and hands were flailing about in a desperate, silent signal to shut them up. What was truly inappropriate was the fact that the patient was under sedation, not a full anaesthetic. There was a very real, very percussive possibility that the patient had heard every single word.

This was the one and only time I have ever seen a lead clinician look like they wanted the floor to swallow them whole. They had to publicly apologise for their unprofessionalism right there in the middle of the OR. It was a stark reminder that the "operating theatre" can be dangerously deceptive.

When I thought this placement could not get any more compelling, I was handed yet another opportunity. I was scheduled to watch a pioneering robot-assisted organ nephrectomy in the morning, followed by a prostatectomy in the afternoon. I had been lucky enough to attend the training session I mentioned earlier, but that had been purely theoretical. It focused on machine operation and technical specs. Now, I was going to see the real thing. The system was nothing short of revolutionary. It was truly astonishing to witness in person.

The mornings scheduled appointments went incredibly well. Even better, my mentor was the lead scrub nurse. As we were prepping, she looked at me and notified me that it was time. I immediately got that specific, electric, feverish feeling where you were unsure whether to be elated or sick. I was up as second scrub. I was officially within the sterile field, and it was up to me. Just me.

My job was to ensure they had every instrument they required. If something was missing, contaminated, or defected, it was my role to anticipate the need. I had to delegate to the circulating team, have the replacement transferred into the field, and prepare it in accordance with strict aseptic guidelines. Thank God I had sat in on that training session. I was at least familiar with the tools: forceps, scissors, cautery tools, and needle holders.

It was relatively quick, lasting a little over two hours. I managed to get through it without passing the wrong instrument or dropping anything. However, the level of concentration required, mainly to ensure I didn't fuck up, left me with a level of exhaustion I had never experienced before or since.

Then came one of my proudest moments. We were cleaning down post-surgery when my mentor walked over and said, "Well done." She was a person of very few words. She was meticulous, thorough, and left no room for error. Coming from her, those two words were a prodigious concession.

Feeling pumped and full of energy, it was on to the afternoon's assembly line. Same robot. Different organ. All performed by a surgeon from their "console in the corner."

It was nicknamed that because of one detail I forgot to mention. Although it was difficult to fathom at first, the consultant was nowhere near the patient. They were totally decoupled from the person on the table. They sat across the room, head buried in a hooded console like a dedicated gamer in a darkened bedroom. They could not see the patient in person and certainly didn't touch them.

The system itself stood over the patient like a giant, multi-limbed spider from a Ridley Scott movie. It had four massive arms draped in clean plastic sleeves, each one holding a tiny, delicate instrument that had been inserted through small ports in the patient's abdomen. Every time the consultant moved their fingers in the console, those massive machine limbs mimicked the motion with a hypnotic fluid grace. It was a virtual procedure, but with very high stakes. For those of you born in the era of PC games and joysticks, it looked as if you were watching someone playing a high-stakes combination of *Pac-Man* with a bit of *Operation* thrown in. Except the graphics were high-definition internal organs and there was no "reset" button if you hit a nerve.

The consultant strode in and headed for their console, clocking me on the way. If I was feeling confident, I would say he was eyeballing me. I looked over my shoulder, fully expecting to see someone much more interesting standing behind me. There was no one. I felt a sudden spike of heat in my cheeks. In the clean, hushed environment of the operating theatre, being noticed by a lead clinician felt like being picked out by a searchlight.

I started to feel a little paranoid, wondering what was going on, when they spoke. "Victoria, right?"

Remember what I said about not shitting yourself? Now was the time to prove I could follow my own advice. "Yes," I replied.

"Good job this morning." "Are you up for circulating for this op?"

"Absolutely," I replied.

"Good, good. Take a handover from the lead scrub and let's see what you've got."

As the circulating nurse, my role had shifted significantly. It was now my job to ensure all documentation, pre, peri, and post-op was completed accurately in real time. I was also responsible for ensuring the team had every piece of equipment and every supply they might need throughout the procedure. I was the glue that ensured the surgery ran smoothly from the moment they started the clock to closing the patient.

We were three-quarters of the way through when a mobile phone started to ping. Everyone panicked. Under no circumstances should you have a mobile phone in the OR, let alone have it switched on. Unless, of course, you are the consultant. Everyone ignored it and the team carried on.

Then, another ping. The consultant called out from behind their console. "Is that mine? I left it next to the computer."

As the circulator, this was my station. I looked at the device and replied, "Yes Sir, it is your phone."

Silence was resumed. At this point, they were cauterising the patient's prostate from the surrounding tissue with finite precision, all while using a joystick. Another ping.

"Victoria, can you check my phone please? Is it a message?"

I quickly scanned the screen and replied, "It is a notification, Sir."

They explained that they were awaiting a message from their child's school. "Victoria, can you check again and make sure it is not the school?"

Blushing was an understatement. I turned desperately to the actual circulator who was there to buffer my total lack of experience with wild eyes showing him the phone screen. All of this whilst trying to hide my complete inability to know what to do. He shrugged his shoulders without uttering a word, a gesture that spoke volumes: This was down to me. Do whatever you need to do. I put my big girl pants on and replied confidently, "It is not the school, Sir. Would you like one of the team to bring it over to you?"

He couldn't touch it, but he could have held the screen up so he could see the notifications for themselves. "That won't be necessary," he muttered.

I was on tenterhooks, praying it wouldn't go off. It did. The phone vibrated on the desk with a buzz that felt like a chainsaw in the silence of the room. Then came the request I was dreading.

"Victoria, tell me who it is. I can't concentrate."

I froze. I felt the weight of every eye in that OR landing squarely on my back. My mentor was still offering me nothing but a blank stare and a sadistic smile that made his eyes shine. I was trapped between a rock and a very unprofessional hard place. Not wanting to be complicit in the person on the table having the wrong organ removed because I was too scared to talk, I tried to play it cool. I replied as diplomatically as possible.

"I think it's personal, Sir. Nothing to worry about."

Their immediate reply took on a far sterner tone. They didn't even look up from the console. Their hands were still dancing on the joysticks, micro-manoeuvring a hot wire inside a human being. "Victoria, please let's not make me ask you again!" I am sure there would have been a "fuck," in there if it hadn't been for circumstance.

The frustration in their voice was the final push I needed. Left with no other choice, and the feeling the structural vibration of my pulse in my throat, I leaned over the phone and read the notification aloud.

"It's Tinder Sir. You have four new matches."

The silence that followed was heavy enough to sink a ship. For two seconds, the only sound was the steady beep-beep-beep of the heart monitor. Then, the consultant let out a short, dry bark of a laugh. They didn't miss a beat with the diathermy cutting through the air with as much precision as the organ he was procuring.

One good thing about face masks was that you could silently piss yourself laughing without anyone seeing your face. I spent the next ten minutes staring intensely at my clipboard, my shoulders shaking, desperately trying to regain my composure.

Despite the dating-app-induced anxiety attack and the cold construction of the compression clamp, the placement was a resounding success. I had performed to specification. It turned out that if you could handle the smell of burning flesh and the ego of a consultant surgeon without passing out, you were halfway to becoming a theatre nurse. I walked away with my head held high, a notebook full of illegible clinical scribbles, and a newfound respect for anyone who spent most of the day staring at a hooded console.

I knew better than to leave without offering a sacrifice to the gods of the clean field. On my final day, I left the team a massive gift box of half decent, high-grade caffeinated coffee. Along with the caffeine, I provided enough biscuits to restock the shelves of a medium-sized food bank. It was a small price to pay for the education I had received. I left the theatres feeling like an honorary member of the tribe, although I was more than happy to return to a world where I was allowed to scratch my own nose whenever I damn well pleased.

11

How to Be a Student Nurse and

Cry When You Need To

The final hurdle. The Stroke Ward. After three years of dragging myself through the trenches of this degree, it felt less like a graduation and more like a parole date. If you count the Access course and the year, I was forced to take out to pull extra shifts to keep a roof over The Boy's head, I'd been at this for four years.

That year out wasn't a "gap year." There were no backpacks or soul-searching in Bali. I was a mercenary in a faded blue tunic. I worked my full-time care assistant hours at the hospital and then spent every free second signed up to a staffing agency that paid practically double if you were willing to travel to the back of beyond while the rest of the world was sleeping or having fun.

I became a connoisseur of the county's B-roads at 4:00 AM. I was fairly certain I had worked in every nursing care home in the area. I knew which ones had the broken lifts, which ones had the "good" biscuits hidden in the staff room, and which ones smelled so strongly of stale urine and industrial lilac that the scent would cling to your hair for three days.

I was a casualty of the system before I had even qualified for it. It was a holding pattern in purgatory: a gruelling twelve-month stretch where the goal wasn't academic excellence: it was financial liquidity. I had to keep a roof over our head. The Rent Book was a financial vice that didn't care about your "passion for nursing." It just wanted feeding. So, I fed it with my spine and my sleep.

My life was a perpetual cycle of Sudocrem and the blue-light hum of the corridors. I learned things they didn't teach you in the lecture theatres: how to de-escalate a resident who thinks you're a thief from the 1940s, how to change a double-bed solo in under three minutes, and how to keep your face undeniably neutral when someone is projectile vomiting on your last clean pair of trousers.

It was dull, repetitive, all-encompassing and eroding. But it was also my armour. When I finally stepped back onto campus to rejoin the world of academia, I wasn't the same wide-eyed student who had started the Access course. I was a veteran of the "grunt work."

That year taught me that nursing wasn't just a career: for people like me, it was a life raft. If I didn't make it through this final placement on the Stroke Ward, there was no safety net. There was the agency bank, the night shifts, and the endless, crushing weight of almost making it.

I walked onto this unit with a bit of a strut. My confidence wasn't a mask for once. I'd spent years as a care assistant in care homes, and stroke patients were my bread and butter. I knew the routine: the thickened fluids that look like wallpaper paste, the meticulous repositioning, and the slow, quiet patience of a morning wash. I was looking forward to seeing the "sharp end" of it. I wanted to be there for the initial rehabilitation, the moment the brain tried to rewire itself like a bombed-out switchboard.

What I wasn't prepared for was the raw, guttural anguish. You see it in the films as a sudden slump followed by a hospital bed, but the reality was a grenade going off in a living room. It wasn't only a clinical event: it was a life being violently dismantled in real time.

There was a specific kind of "living grief" that haunted a Stroke Ward. It was the sight of a spouse looking at their partner of forty-odd years and realising the person who once knew the neurological blueprint of their own autonomy, was trapped behind a wall of aphasia and confusion.

The families were the hardest part. They looked at us with this desperate, wide-eyed expectation, convinced that we had a magic pill in the cupboard that would un-clot the brain and reset the clock to just before nine. They thought medicine was a light switch. They didn't want to hear about the "complexities of recovery" or "neuroplasticity." They wanted their parent back.

Watching that disbelief sink in was like watching a controlled demolition go wrong. You saw the moment the penny dropped; it hit them that the road back wasn't a week of antibiotics: it was a brutal, uphill crawl through a thicket of physical therapy and frustration. The light at the end of my tunnel was shining brightly, but for the people in those beds, the lights had been smashed out.

Then I met my mentor. She was young. Not just "early in her career" young, but biologically offensive young. They had bypassed 'A' Levels, sprinted through an Access course, and qualified at twenty-two. By the time I met them, they were just shy of twenty-three and already being groomed for a Junior Charge Nurse role.

Usually, that kind of rapid ascent smells like clinical arrogance or a lack of real-world seasoning, but they were the real deal. After our first preliminary interview, I wasn't intimidated. I was impressed. They were knowledgeable, professional, and possessed a level of self-assurance that usually takes a decade to cultivate. Most importantly, they were excited. They had an infectious, unbridled energy for the job that I thought had been beaten out of the profession years ago.

They saw me not as a pair of hands to help with the turns, but as a protégé. They actively hunted for opportunities for me, dragging me into rooms to witness clinical competencies I didn't even know existed. They pushed me beyond the stale tick-boxes of the university curriculum. Their attitude was a refreshing, high-voltage jolt to my system.

I also had to eat my words. I previously went on record saying it was impossible to look anything other than a collapsed tent while wearing a nursing uniform. I was wrong. They had the aesthetic down to a fine art. Their hair was always scraped into a deliberately messy low knot that obeyed the laws of physics and humidity. Their makeup was light, expertly applied, and still somehow stayed in perfect situ under the soul-sucking fluorescent lights of the unit.

Most impressively, they never looked knackered. We would be at the tail end of a brutal thirteen-hour shift, surrounded by the smell of the suffocating aroma of biological surrender, and they would still look like they had just stepped out of a salon. I, meanwhile, usually looked physiologically spent and like I had been sat on by a patient.

There was a lot to be said for the wisdom of experience, but there was also a specific, vital power in enthusiasm. She was walking the path I was currently hacking through with a machete, and for the first time in four years, she made me feel like the destination might be worth the trip.

Then came the shift that would end up as one of the most emotionally harrowing experiences of my entire journey. It started like any other midweek shift. The only slight difference was the weight of the invisible pips on my shoulders. My mentor had decided it was time to take the stabilisers off. They entrusted me to run the shift solo, stepping back into a support role while I took the lead.

Handover was a blur of neurological observations and bowel movements. Once the clipboard was officially mine, I was assigned a bay of six patients. I had developed a morning ritual that I guarded fiercely: I introduced myself to every single patient before I touched a tablet or a thermometer.

Not every nurse does this. Some treat the patients like tasks on a to-do list, a series of obstructed airways and leaking cannulas. I found that even five seconds of actual human eye contact put people at ease. It built a therapeutic relationship faster than any clinical somatic, even if I was moving at a sprint.

On a busy ward, speed is the only currency that matters. Patients are admitted, transferred, or discharged in a dizzying cycle of musical beds. It is not unheard of to have your entire bay flipped three times in a single shift. You start the day with six elderly men and end it with six women, wondering where the time went and which one of them was "Nil by Mouth."

But one lady stood out. Jodie.

As soon as I approached her bed, she greeted me with a smile that felt like a warm radiator in a cold house. She reached out and took my hand in hers, a gesture of trust that caught me off guard. She welcomed me to care for her, telling me she was grateful I was there and that she looked forward to getting to know me over the shift.

I felt a rare spark of genuine optimism. That day was going to be a good day. I had my mentor's trust, a patient who appeared to like me, and an extra bonus that felt like a gift from the nursing gods: Mumma Bear was my assigned healthcare assistant.

You remember Mumma Bear? She was the friend who had literally kept me alive during the darkest parts of the degree, the one who ran the hot baths, let me crash in her spare room, and fed me when I was too broken to hold a fork. Having her in my bay felt like having a tactical advantage. We were a team. We were invincible. Or so I thought.

Jodie had been dealt a hand that would have made a professional gambler fold and walk away. Months ago, in her mid-fifties, she'd been diagnosed with advanced ovarian cancer. The "Big C" hadn't just knocked on her door: it had kicked it in. She'd endured a radical surgery and enough chemotherapy to make her feel like her blood was made of battery acid.

Despite the exhaustion, she refused to stay in bed. She sat up in her chair, defiant, as if lying down was an admission of defeat she wasn't ready to sign.

Before the world collapsed, Jodie had been a whirlwind. She owned a café, spent her days baking, and managed a catering company on the side. When she wasn't covered in flour, she was an avid activist, raising money for charity through running, more running, and then, for good measure, a bit more running. Her personal best for a 10k was under an hour. Most people half her age couldn't manage that without a literal tailwind and a motorised scooter.

Now, she was of a very slight build. I couldn't help but notice the cruel, obvious muscle wastage. Her face was gaunt, her skin sallow, and her eyes had that sunken, weary look that comes from fighting a war on two fronts.

But she was still beautiful. She wore a brightly coloured silk scarf wrapped around her bald head like a crown, a matching caftan, and perfectly manicured nails. "Important to look good until the end" was her mantra. It wasn't about vanity: it was about dignity. It was the only part of her life she still had a firm grip on.

The latest blow had been a one-sided neurological infarction. In the medical world, we call it a Cerebrovascular Accident, which is a polite way of saying her brain had suffered a catastrophic plumbing failure. Most people would have crumbled, but Jodie considered herself lucky.

She viewed her one-sided weakness as a minor inconvenience rather than a tragedy.

"I can still walk, talk, eat, and drink independently," she told me with a wink. "If that's not a win, I don't know what is. I still shit myself occasionally, but then, who doesn't?"

It was the kind of gallows humour that nurses thrive on. It made the unbearable parts of the job feel human. She was a runner who could barely stand, a baker who was currently being served hospital rice pudding, and yet she was the most positive person in the bay. Looking at her, I felt that familiar, dangerous spark of hope. I should have known better.

A little after midday, the call bell above Jodie's bed chimed. It was a polite, rhythmic sound, unlike the frantic, staccato bursts of the more demanding patients. Mumma Bear went to investigate and returned to me almost immediately with a look on her face that I knew meant a deviation from the care plan.

"Victoria," she said, her voice dropping to a conspiratorial whisper. "We've got a special request."

I followed her over to the bay. It turned out Jodie's only son was visiting that afternoon, and the stakes for this meeting were sky-high. He had finished a First-Class Honours Law Degree from an elite university: the kind of achievement that usually warrants a brass band and a parade. He was taking a year out before disappearing into the soul-crushing machinery of a legal career, and the next day, he was set to fly out for a year long trip around the world.
Jodie looked at me with those sunken, hopeful eyes. "Is there any way we could do a little something special for him?"

"Of course," I replied, the words leaving my mouth before my brain could calculate the logistics. "Leave it with us."

I cleared it with my mentor, who gave me a supportive nod, and then I set about trying to "work some magic." In hospital terms, magic usually requires a budget, and trying to get petty cash voucher out of the Service was like trying to extract blood from a very dry stone. The only time I had ever successfully requisitioned funds was for a taxi voucher to shift a delayed discharge and free up a bed. Asking for a "celebration budget" for a dying woman's son would have been laughed out of the finance office.

I reached into my bag and pulled out my wallet. I found a twenty-pound note. I categorically could not afford to lose that twenty pounds: it was petrol money, school shoe money, survival money. But some things are more important than a balanced ledger.

I handed the cash to Mumma Bear and told her to get whatever she could to decorate the bed space. She didn't just meet the brief: she annihilated it. She'd gone down to the site shop, told the assistant exactly what we were doing, and came trotting back onto the unit with banners, balloons, and a box of muffins. To top it off, she handed me a tenner in change. Even the shop staff, it seemed, weren't immune to Jodie's story.

We set to work, turning a stark, clinical bed space into something that looked, for a fleeting moment, like a home. It was a tiny island of midnight-blue pride in a sea of beige vinyl and ailment.

The bed space looked like a five-year-old's birthday party. It was garish, loud, and wrong on almost every level, yet it was exactly what we needed. For a few hours, the ward felt different. Jodie sat in her chair, a queen in a silk scarf, sipping fizzy pop from a plastic cup with her husband and her son. We couldn't risk real wine: the Modern

Matron would have had a cerebrovascular event of her own if she'd caught us: so we made do with the sugary, bubbling substitute.

They laughed. They talked about university and the world beyond the site car park. From the nursing station, I watched them, clinging to the illusion that this was a normal family having a normal celebration.

The second the door swung shut behind them, the illusion shattered.

Jodie didn't cry, she broke. She began sobbing with a raw, uncontrollable grief that seemed to vibrate through the thin hospital curtains. I approached her bed tentatively. In nursing, you spend a lot of time gauging the silence, trying to decide if a patient needs a hand to hold or the dignity of being left alone. Jodie made the choice for me. She reached out and patted the edge of her mattress, beckoning me to sit.

"Oh Victoria," she choked out, her voice thin and ragged. "He doesn't know it, but that was the last time I will ever see him. There is no more treatment. I've got less than a few months."

I was floored. I couldn't even manage a platitude. I sat there, my mouth probably slightly agape, as the weight of her secret pressed down on the room. She took my hands, her grip surprisingly firm for someone so frail.

"If he knew, he wouldn't go," she whispered. Her eyes were searching for my soul, desperate for me to understand. "I would rather see him chase his dreams. I want to hear about the memories he's making before I die. I want to take those stories with me."

The professionalism I had spent three years cultivating evaporated. I thought of The Boy. I thought of the lengths to which I would go to protect his future, the way I had slaved through that wilderness year to keep his world steady. The tears came. Hot and impossible to stop. Sometimes, the textbooks told you to maintain a clinical distance, but the textbooks weren't there in the late afternoon on a midweek shift when a mother was choosing her son's joy over her own goodbye. Sometimes, it was okay to cry with your patients. It was the only honest response left.

When I turned up for my next shift, the bed was empty. The banners were gone. The balloons had been deflated and tossed into the clinical waste. Jodie had been transferred to a hospice during the night. I felt a sharp, gut-wrenching pain in my chest. I hadn't said goodbye. I had been so busy being a student nurse that I'd forgotten how quickly the exit door could swing shut.

***

Next up came a dreaded run of night shifts. There was a specific kind of madness that set in around the third night: a surreal, heavy-lidded fatigue where the ward lights felt too bright and the silence felt like a physical responsibility.

One night stayed with me, not because of a clinical crisis or a patient in distress, but because of a colleague. When I started this journey, I assumed the stress would come from the trauma of the patients. I didn't realise I would also have to navigate the "bullying game" played by fellow nurses. Bullying in nursing felt like a juxtaposition. It was a total oxymoron. How could a profession built on the foundation of compassion house people who took pleasure in breaking their own? This experience taught me exactly how it happened, and more importantly, how to survive it.

It was after four, the hour where the soul feels thinnest. I was hunkered down at the computer desk at the central nursing station, completing my notes. The station sat in the middle of the ward, an "open office" in theory, but I was tucked away in a cubby hole behind the wall that housed the status board. I was deep in the "Twilight Zone," documenting the lives of seven different patients, when I was approached by a new student.

She sat down next to me without saying a word. Out of the corner of my eye, I watched her. She wasn't doing paperwork. She wasn't checking the board. She was just sitting there, turned toward me, vibrating with a silent, awkward tension.

I put down my pen. "Are you alright?" I asked.

A long pause followed. Her expression shifted into a strained, internal frown, the kind of look someone wears when they are crying behind their eyes. Finally, she spoke. "I'm really struggling."

I gave her a nudge. I told her I knew the road was tough and that I'd been exactly where she was. With a bit of encouragement, the dam finally broke. It wasn't the clinical side that was drowning her: it was the learning logs and reflections. The "invisible" work.

I had seen many brilliant students fail because of this. They had a natural bedside manner, they could interpret diagnostics like a pro, and they were hotshots at clinical skills, yet they were slaughtered by the documentation. They could save a life in the small hours but couldn't write a comprehensive reflection on it at 4am.

Do you remember when I asked if nursing should be an academic degree? This was why. We were losing good, compassionate people to the god of the "Practice Assessment Portfolio." The system was designed to produce academics who could cite a paper, even if they couldn't handle a bedpan without gagging.

I decided to take her under my wing. I told her I needed to finish up two records, and then, if she grabbed her portfolio, we could sacrifice our short break to sit and go through a few points together. She didn't just walk she trotted off at high speed, returning seconds later with her heavy folder tucked under one arm and two cups of black instant coffee. This wasn't the artisanal stuff from the site foyer. This was ward coffee: a liquid so dark and viscous that your teaspoon could practically stand up in it. It was the kind of caffeine that doesn't wake you up: it reverberates your internal organs.

We set ourselves up in our little cubby hole. I started sifting through the work she had already completed, asking her to pinpoint the areas where she felt like she was drowning. We quickly identified the culprits. She didn't lack intelligence: she lacked clarity and the ability to write concisely. She was trying to tell a story when The university wanted a forensic report.

Heads down and speaking in hushed tones to avoid waking the patients in the middle bay, we started to build a plan. I was a "work smart, not hard" kind of person. By year two, I had already hacked through the dense thicket of academia she was entering. I had struggled with the exact same hurdles, so I shared the structure I had developed to keep my head above water.

It was a simple four-step process that I applied to every single entry. It was designed to cut out the "fluff," eliminate colloquial language, and create a short but comprehensive evidence-based log (with at least one reference). It turned an hour-long agonising session into a twenty-minute clinical task.

She looked at me like I had performed a miracle. Her expression was the same one a new student wears when they see a perfect hospital corner executed for the first time: pure, unadulterated awe. With a surge of excitement that cut right through the around-half-four fatigue, she asked if I could help her write one right there and then.

"Sure thing," I said, ignoring the dull ache in my own lower back. I knew that helping her wasn't only about the paperwork. It was about making sure the system didn't chew her up and spit her out before she even got her registration.

As we were huddled over the portfolio, the Senior Charge Nurse on shift returned to the unit. They had been absent for hours. Where they actually went during the night was anyone's guess, considering there were no management meetings, and the rest of the site was running on a skeleton crew. They couldn't use the usual excuse of being "stuck in a briefing."

They were clearly pissed off with wherever they had been. They stormed onto the ward with an air of self-importance that they hadn't yet earned. They expected the Red Sea to part and the staff to stand to attention, but they lacked the actual presence of a Matron. Consequently, no one moved. We all kept doing our jobs.

Marching behind the nursing station, they decided to make their presence felt by shouting at us. "You too need to shut up! If you have to speak, do it quietly. Patients are trying to sleep!"

The irony was thick enough to choke on. She was the only person in the building currently behaving like a megaphone. Both of us raised our heads, preparing to offer a feigned, tired apology. Before we could even draw breath to explain, she was gone. All we saw were her heels stomping off the unit, leaving a trail of destruction and a very awake, very "Mad Doris" in their wake.

Nearing handover, during the grey, miserable hour before the morning brief, she returned in full force. The moment they laid eyes on me, they launched into an erratic rant.

194

"Under no circumstances should you be idly talking on a night shift," she hissed. "Patients need sleep."

I tried to keep my voice level. I tried to explain that I wasn't discussing a weekend out on the piss: I was assisting a fellow student with the clinical reflections they needed to pass their placement. They cut me off before I could finish the sentence.

"Have I not told you before to shut up?"

They were fully oblivious to the fact that, on their way to berate us, they had walked past a huddle of care assistants who were watching *Love Island* on a mobile phone and laughing out loud. They hadn't noticed them. They only had eyes for the students. It seemed they had a specific, centrifugal appetite for berating the people at the bottom of the food chain.

The exhaustion of four years of struggle finally hit a breaking point. My filter failed. I threw out a flippant comment as they turned to leave. "You don't need to teach me to suck eggs," I said, the sarcasm dripping off the words like warm honey.

They hightailed it off the ward, but the second the words left my mouth, an overarching sense of dread washed over me. I had let my just-before-handover brain take the wheel. I tried to console myself with the idea that they were so busy being a bitch that they probably hadn't heard me. I was wrong. I had been too loud, and I was most definitely within earshot. I just didn't know it yet.

This was the moment every student nurse feared. It was the sudden, cold transition from being a clinical asset to being a "problem" on a spreadsheet. In the world of the NHS, a "Concern Flag" was the professional equivalent of a black spot on a pirate's map.

I was now going to introduce you to something that was, quite honestly, a nurse's worst nightmare. I called it the DE. This, my friends, was the Dreaded Email. You would hear far more about this later in this trilogy, but for now, note that this was any email you absolutely did not want to receive. Ever. It was the digital equivalent of a cold hand on the back of your neck.

This was my first. It arrived from university, sitting in my inbox like an unexploded bomb. The subject line was three words long, but they carried enough weight to sink a ship: "Cause for Concern."

WTF?

I sat there staring at the screen blankly. Time seemed to warp and stretch, for what felt like an eternity. I went over every possible scenario in my head. I thought about The Boy, the five years of struggle, the staffing agency shifts, and the petrol money. I thought about the finish line I was so close to crossing. Then, I hit the open key.

I had been reported.

They hadn't just heard my flippant comment: they had weaponised it. I had been officially reported to university for insubordination. Apparently, telling a senior nurse not to teach me how to suck eggs was enough to trigger a formal review into my professional conduct.

In a world where patients are dying of neglect and wards are crumbling, this person had found the time to write a formal document because their ego had been bruised before handover. It was petty. It was vindictive. And because they held the power of a Senior Charge Nurse over my head, it was potentially life-altering.

The "Cause for Concern Flag" process was designed to be a supportive measure, or so the handbook claimed. In reality, it felt like being called into the headmaster's office while the rest of the school watched. It was a stain on your record before you'd even earned the right to have a record. I felt a sick, hollow sensation in the pit of my stomach. I had survived the wilderness year and the heartbreak of the stroke ward, only to be taken down by a metaphor about poultry products.

The process of Fitness to Practice was something I wouldn't wish on my worst enemy. Personally or professionally, it was soul-destroying, mentally draining, and nothing short of debilitating. It was the clinical equivalent of being placed in the stocks in the middle of the town square while your peers were invited to throw stones at your competence.

This was my first brush with the blunt instrument of professional judgment. Because it was handled by university and not a national regulatory body, it was technically the "lite" version of the nightmare. It was a mere dress rehearsal for the real, life-altering trauma that would come years later once I was registered: a period of my life so dark and predatory that it remained the most harrowing thing I have ever endured. But even this junior version was enough to make my hands shake.

I was lucky. My Academic Advisor was one of the most caring individuals I had ever had the pleasure of meeting. They didn't look at me like a criminal: they looked at me like a tired mother who was four years deep into what should have been a three-year .

The meeting took place in a barren office that smelled of old paper and anxiety. It began with the standard opening. "So then, Victoria, in your own words, tell me what happened?"

I didn't lie. I didn't have the energy for a cover-up. "It was the small hours of the morning," I said, my voice flat with residual exhaustion. "I was in the twilight zone. I was approached by a fellow student asking for help with their documentation. We were discussing it in hushed tones when the Senior Charge Nurse decided we were idly gossiping and reprimanded us. I don't like being told to shut up. I allowed my fatigue to get the better of me and I told them they didn't need to teach me to suck eggs. I said it a little louder than I should have."

My advisor sat there for a moment, their face a mask of academic neutrality. Then, I saw their chest hitch. They were stifling laughter. The sheer, petty absurdity of a senior lead filing a "Cause for Concern" over an old idiom about eggs was clearly not lost on them.

They signed off the paperwork right there. No case to answer. The only feedback I received was delivered with a sympathetic, knowing smile.

"Next time, Victoria, think it. For the love of God, don't say it out loud. Remember the Code and if you get asked the same question in the future reflect on your choice of words and don't say you'd do it again, only quieter."

I walked out of that office feeling a massive weight lift, but the seed of distrust had been planted. I recognised then that the "Nursing Family" wasn't always a support system. Sometimes, it was a firing squad.

***

This was it. The stroke ward was the actual emergency medicine I had dreamed about experiencing since the first day. These were the life-and-death situations that felt like they belonged in a television drama, not in the daily life of a woman who had spent the last four years measuring her existence in the price of a pint of milk and the hours of sleep she could steal before the school run.

Thrombolysis was the high-stakes gamble of the medical world. It involved using "clot-busting" medications to chemically dissolve the blockages in a patient's brain during the golden hour of a neuro emergency. If you got it right, you could watch someone regain the use of their limbs in real time. If it went wrong, the risks were catastrophic. My "satellite" placement with the team was a sensory overload of adrenaline and professional precision. It had everything: the static-heavy crackle of first-responder radios, the blur of rapid assessment, and the frantic, coordinated dance of urgent treatment. I stood in the middle of A&E as the red phone rang, signalling a "Neuro Alert" incoming.

I watched the aircraft descend onto the landing pad, the rotors whipping up a gale that seemed to echo the chaos in my own chest. I wasn't observing from the sidelines anymore. I was part of the emergency response team. I was the one holding the clipboard, checking the onset times, and prepping the infusion pumps.

It was the ultimate "Tonal Whiplash." One day I was being bullied for mentoring a junior, and the next I was standing on the frontline of human survival, watching the best in the business save a brain from melting.

As I completed my final shift, I accepted that the "Student Nurse" label was finally, mercifully, falling away. I looked at the sign-off in my Practice Assessment Portfolio. My mentor's signature was the final key in the lock of a five-year prison cell.
I thought about the wilderness year. I thought about the staffing agency shifts and the smell of industrial lilac in the care homes. I thought about the £20 I had spent on muffins and banners for a dying

woman's son. Every mile on the flickering fuel light, every tear shed in a site car park, and every "Suck Eggs" comment had led to this.

I walked out of the hospital doors and into the cool evening air. I wasn't the same woman who had started this journey. I was tired, yes. I was cynical, certainly. But as I headed home to The Boy, I knew one thing for certain: I was a Nurse.

The bang wasn't just the sound of an aircraft landing. It was the sound of my old life ending and my real career finally beginning.

12

How to Be a Student Nurse and

Take the Stabilisers Off

Nursing degree: done. Whilst I could bore you with the finalities of sign off assessments, paperwork and all the tick box exercises you must endure to prove that you have navigated the labyrinth successfully and remain standing, this chapter is dedicated to summarising the experience into a snapshot of the future.

As your nursing career progresses you will begin to realise that the many, valiant nurses that have paved the way you are about to embark on have developed a distinct glossary of terminologies, labels and identifiers for some of the most exhilarating and soul crushing elements of what donning the blue uniform and holding your registration primarily entails.

I learnt many of these along the way but as a student failed to recognise them and most certainly didn't possess the tool kit I required to stay alive and sane. So, this is my recap of the student experience with the knowledge and hindsight they don't teach you when you become in my case Unique Identifier UI001.

There is a moment on most shifts when the ward sounds like a kettle about to boil. Machines sing in alternating keys, the phone insists it has rights, and your tea has become that special temperature that only exists in hospitals: the temperature of regret. In that noise, it is easy to fold into silence. I used to do that. Silence felt like control, but it was a weight that grew heavier every hour. Survival starts small: one hand on the bench or the rail. Breathe in for a count of four and out for six. Brief the next step out loud. Begin again. It's not poetry: it's a safety plan you can run on any corridor.

Nursing taught me to face hard truths gently. We care for people who carry hidden harm and work beside colleagues who carry heavy stories home in the boot with the scrubs and a sandwich that has merged with a latex glove. Kindness is not a soft option here: it is a skill with muscle. Facing hard truths gently means presence, boundaries, and policy. Notice what does not sit right. Name the concern to the right person. Navigate using the safeguarding pathway you have, not the one you wish the machine had written with due care and diligence.

This is not about dramatic reveals: it is about small, steady acts that keep patients safe and keep you whole. Nurses are over twice as likely to experience domestic abuse than the general population. It is not a statistic to scroll past with a shrug and a grim smile. If you are the one carrying this, you are not alone. Speak to someone. Find your person. Strength is not silence: that sentence sits in your pocket with your ID and your favourite pen. If today is loud, start small.

Every new nurse feels it: that burning desire to leap from observation to action. You are fuelled by textbook knowledge, excited by the challenge, and frankly, tired of standing in the corner. You want to run. You want to apply the complex dressings and draw up the medicines, yet you hear the word "Observe" so often you think it is your new job title. Your legs are ready to walk the walk, not just talk the talk, but your seniors deliver the clear demand: "Walk first". That mandate to master the fundamentals before seeking independence is not a punishment: it is the single most important safety lesson you will ever receive.

Walking first is precision in slow motion. You learn the methodical checks that everyone pretends are obvious, the ones that even experienced clinicians must deliberately recall under pressure. You must rein in your enthusiasm and take one step at a time even if you could do it in your sleep. To understand why this slow-paced mentorship is non-negotiable, we must look at the data. Research indicates that a shocking 48 to 52 percent of newly qualified nurses report making a medication or treatment error in their first year or so. Rushing is the fastest path to joining that statistic.

Watching is not passive: it is training with the safety guard on. Eyes first means you watch like a teammate, not a tourist, tracking the calm order beneath the noise. When you can accurately narrate a task back to your mentor, your hands are ready to step in. Hands later, is how muscle memory develops in the right direction. If you are ready but your mentor is hesitant, use a professional communication strategy to bridge the trust gap. Flatter with facts. Acknowledge their focus on safety, state the facts about your review of the policy, and ask confidently to lead the task under close observation. You are earning the experience by providing evidential proof of your competence. Your speed today matters less than your safety tomorrow.

For the student nurse pursuing a degree while battling financial precarity, juggling minimum wage work, full-time placements, and the relentless pressure of bills, being skint is a lifestyle. The cost of this degree is measured in more than tuition fees: it is measured in lost sleep, skipped meals, and the immense weight of knowing there is no financial safety net. This struggle demands an exceptional level of resilience that ultimately forges an incredibly capable nurse, the kind who can manage an emergency while surviving purely on the bare minimum of sustenance.

Your survival strategy must become as precise as your Safe Medicate calculations. The harsh reality is that the student loan is barely a stretched-thin resource. It is not a salary: it is more like a stingy relative who shows up once a term, gives you an envelope of cash that smells faintly of mothballs, and then vanishes, leaving you to manage for months. To survive, you must treat your budget like a high-risk patient chart. Audit every expense and track every pound to ensure there are no unexpected haemorrhages.

When you are skint, your time is the most expensive, non-renewable resource you possess. You are running on empty, and you certainly cannot afford the luxury of passive learning. Success hinges on exploiting the "Flashcard Fragment": those five, ten, or fifteen-minute pockets of time that usually go to waste. This is where you conduct the Two-Minute Drill. Before opening any notes, set a two-minute timer and aggressively write down everything you can recall about the last topic on a blank page. The panic of the timer is a more effective memory stimulant than the gentle prodding of a mentor

When the exhaustion sets in, you need a clear reminder of the payoff. This degree is a strategic, high-value investment. The nursing degree is the turning point that forever separates your past financial insecurity from your future professional stability. You are securing a life where an unexpected car repair does not signal the apocalypse.

Starting a new clinical placement is always an exercise in controlled chaos. But try starting one where the placement lead introduces you not as a student, but as the continuation of a decades-long legend. Being told you are there to continue your relative's legacy is enough to make you want the floor to open up and swallow you whole. Every student nurse, whether they realise it or not, is fighting a Legacy Battle. You are constantly measured against a clinical lead, a social media icon, or the ghost of the perfect First-Class Honours student who rotated through recently. The pressure to be a sequel is immense, but the world needs you, not a cheap replica.

When your history precedes you, you quickly realise you are being studied. Every hesitation or question is scrutinised and amplified, creating a scrutiny culture that breeds crippling self-doubt. Around two-thirds of professionals' experience Impostor Syndrome. That terrifying feeling that everyone is about to realise you have no idea what you are doing is a sign that you are invested in succeeding, not failing. To survive, you must filter the noise. Gossip is distraction, but formal feedback is regulatory capital.

Build a strict, two-tier system for processing information. High priority currency is the documented assessment criteria and formal mentor feedback. Low priority noise is everything else: the nostalgic anecdotes about how your predecessors would have done it, the prejudicial dissection, and the gossip.

Discard the noise immediately. When you are under scrutiny, use a tactical communication strategy to force the conversation back to your present competence. Use the expectation redirect script when someone starts a comparison. Say: "Thank you, I hope to reach that level one day. But right now, I am working on mastering this specific skill. Could you watch me do this task and tell me if I handled it correctly according to current policy?". This turns subjective comparison into objective feedback. Establishing professional autonomy is the biggest fight of your student career. You are the origin story.

Sometimes the hardest module isn't clinical: it is Emotional Survival 101. Imagine starting Day One of university a week after a traumatic, volatile relationship breakdown. Suddenly, you are faced with the crushing dichotomy of walking into a clinical placement and pretending to be a functional, engaged human being while internally you are screaming. This is the reality of being single, lonely, and desperately trying to appear happy while the world feels like it is collapsing.

The first thing you learn is how to wear two uniforms. The first is your professional exterior: competent, caring, and stable. The second is your inner self: grieving, terrified, and emotionally exhausted. Allowing the inner mess to compromise the outer uniform is not an option because patient safety and your academic success depend on your ability to perform. This demands Radical Compartmentalisation.

When the internal chaos threatens to spill out, you must practice the mental exercise of leaving the emotional wreckage at the door. Imagine placing the trauma into a physical box and locking it in your bag or your locker. Tell yourself: "I will pick this up at the end of the shift. Right now, I belong to the patient". You are earning the right to fall apart later.

Statistical validation tells us that around one in five nursing students report experiencing symptoms of depression or anxiety. If you feel emotionally exhausted, you are not failing, you are a statistic. To survive, you must use Observational Participation: the skill of being functionally present without being emotionally exposed. Engage on the surface regarding the weather or assignment stress but understand that superficial level connection and engagement is sufficient for your psychological safety right now.

The mask must come down for a few minutes to prevent a system crash. We call this The Decompression Pocket. Find a strict, private space: a locked toilet cubicle, the secure room, or a quiet stairwell. Spend the time on one core action: slow, deliberate breathing, a brief cry, or a candid voice note to a trusted person. You can't be a healer if you're haemorrhaging empathy. Grant grace to the student you are now for the messy tears and the grades that aren't perfect scores.

When we discuss acute care nursing, we often focus on the clinical triumphs or the technical complexities of the role. However, a different reality emerges defined by what I call the sensory assault. High acuity environments are high velocity spaces fuelled by cortisol, urgency, and the constant hum of life sustaining technology. For a student nurse, the transition into this space can feel like a vertical climb.

To understand why nurses, feel so overwhelmed, we must look at the structural reality of the NHS. Currently, the machine operates with approximately 2.3 hospital beds per 1,000 people. When compared to the international average of roughly 4.6, the discrepancy is staggering. We are effectively managing a national health crisis with near half of the physical infrastructure of our international peers. This 2.3 Factor is the engine behind the sensory overload. It creates an environment where the music never stops and the contestants are always the most vulnerable. This is why you feel internally vibration long after your shift has ended. It is not a personal failure of resilience: it is a physiological response to a system that has exceeded its capacity.

In these high-pressure settings, the teaching philosophy often reverts to the traditional model of see one, do one. This rapid immersion often forces students to mask their uncertainty to avoid being seen as a liability. One of the most difficult reflections involves the toxic reputation that can plague certain services. I recall an instance where a unit was rebranded from an MAU to an AMU: they didn't change the culture only the order of the acronym and hoped the bullying would stop noticing. A bit like putting lipstick on a pig.

How do we survive this assault? You must perform an SBAR on yourself. Before you walk through your front door, assess your own vitals.

Situation: shift finished, battery dead.

Background: the unit was on full escalation.

Assessment: sympathy tank is bone dry. Profound somatic restlessness present.

Recommendation: immediate, radical decompression. Choose a vice: one that can't potentially kill you if you overindulge.

Your compassion tank is not infinite, and resilience should not be a badge of honour worn to justify systemic failure. You cannot pour from a shattered cup.

The narrative shifts away from the clinical chaos of the wards and into the quiet, fluorescent lit corridors of university. This is not about a medical emergency: it is about a different kind of trauma called moral injury. It occurs when the institutions responsible for our education fail to uphold the very values they teach. From the first week of training, we are programmed to look past the surface of human behaviour. We are taught that aggression is often fear, and that boundary breaking is frequently a cry for help. We are trained to lead with empathy and maintain a professional mask at all costs.

However, during my later year, I discovered the dark side of this conditioning. When I became the target of persistent and unwanted advances from a peer, my nursing brain took over. Instead of feeling the righteous anger needed for self-protection, I instinctively moved into care mode. I found myself acting as a pro bono therapist for the person who was harassing me. I was gaslighting my own instincts because I had been taught that being a good nurse meant being infinitely accepting.

When I finally broke through that conditioning and decided to speak up, I was met with a masterclass in institutional reality attrition. I walked into the university administration office expecting a solution but I was told that the person who targeted me had a bright future that I should consider. I was asked to carry the weight of their career on my shoulders while my own safety was treated as a secondary concern. The message was clear: the reputation of the institution mattered more than the safety of the individual student. I walked out of that office feeling like a ghost in my own career.

We were being taught the importance of speaking truth to power while power was being used to ensure a student stayed silent. Resilience cannot fix a toxic culture. Empathy is a nurse's greatest tool, but without boundaries, it becomes a weapon used to silence us.

Moving into Community nursing is a masterclass in clinical adaptability. It marks the transition from the rigid structure of the ward to the raw, unpredictable reality of the road. This is the Autonomy Paradox: the jarring shift from being a highly monitored student to a practitioner trusted to fly solo in an environment no university can control. Every student eventually hits an invisible ceiling where your skills are sharp, but you are suddenly pulled back into observe only mode. Lancing the boil of this clinical resentment requires more than just keeping your head down: it requires a tactical shift in how we perceive student capability.

When you leave the ward, you lose the safety of the controlled environment. You are no longer working in a sanitised space: you are a guest in the patient's world. One hour might be spent in an environment that feels like a wrecked flat, redressing wounds amidst debris and drug paraphernalia. The next is spent in an opulent home with marble floors and award-winning gardens. The unvarnished truth of Community nursing is that clinical standards must remain identical regardless of the area or the state of the living room floor.

Because the community environment is so raw, the sensory and emotional debt can be immense. You witness realities, from neglected children to the anguish of poverty, that a textbook cannot prepare you for. My mentor taught me the Art of Recalibration: the necessity of finding a neutral space after a high stakes encounter. Sitting on a public bench for a few minutes in silence is not a luxury: it is a professional requirement to ensure you don't carry the weight of the last address into the next one.

The ultimate turning point is the solo flight. Being handed a route-ordered patient list, signing the travel agreement, and being told "see you when you get back" is the most significant validation a student can receive. When you are flying solo, you stop performing nursing and start living it. Validation is a clinical requirement: when a student is trusted with autonomy, they rise to meet it.

In the clinical world, we are taught to fear the Never Ever Event. But as a student nurse, I encountered a different kind of professional threat: the moment a high performing clinical practitioner is nearly derailed by the inflexible world of the Academic Matrix. Decoding this matrix reveals that nursing academia often values your ability to reference over your ability to rescue. It is a world where your independent thoughts on patient safety are often secondary to what a researcher wrote years ago. I had to learn a new skill called Strategic Compliance.

I recall my first major assignment with a mixture of pride and bitterness. My clinical score was ninety-eight per cent, but my academic paper passed by exactly three marks. I was labelled a borderline case. It felt like an assassination of my professional character. I had to learn to delete my personality and feed the markers exactly what they craved: buzzwords, theory blending, and perfect bibliographies. We need to stop the shame associated with the borderline pass. In the university nursing degree, around forty per cent is the hero of the story.

Perfectionism is a luxury that the modern student nurse often cannot afford. When you are balancing long bank shifts as a care assistant alongside full-time placements, your capacity for academic excellence is hampered by the physiological need for survival. Your registration does not come with a grade transcript printed on the back. The ward only asks if you are safe and if your code of conduct is tolerable. Treat academic feedback like a pathology report: strip away the emotion and look for the clinical requirements needed to pass.

Strategic compliance is about protecting your energy for where it matters most: the bedside. If the matrix demands you quote a specific theorist to prove you can change a dressing, then you find that quote and move on. You are not failing the profession by refusing to be an academic superstar: you are succeeding by ensuring you reach the finish line. A pass is a win, and every win brings you one step closer to the registration that really counts.

Every placement becomes an oracle of all knowledge: an environment where the hierarchy is so steep it feels like a tonnage. Being in the presence of a senior clinicians is a volatile mix of adoration and fear. In these environments learning the art of being able to professionally challenge effectively can be the difference between catching a medication error and filling out a coroner's report. Your career or a prison cell.

You aren't there to be "nice" and "compliant." You are there to be the final barrier between a patient and a catastrophe. If a consultant who has more letters after their name than a patients discharge summary has spelling mistakes is about to prescribe a dose of Gentamicin that would liquify a patient's kidneys, you have to speak up.

The system loves the language of safety; it prints it on lanyards and plasters it across the staff room walls in primary colours. It tells you that Patient Safety is the north star, a collective responsibility that transcends the petty boundaries of grade and ego. But the machinery isn't built for safety. It is built for Systemic Preservation. When you spot the error, when you see the "Consultant's Oversight" for the impending fatality it could be, you aren't just checking a dose; you are sticking a crowbar into the gears of an ancient, pride heavy machine. Systemic Failure is rarely a simple. Catastrophic explosion. It is a slow, quiet rot of "minor" omissions and "common" practices that everyone sees but no one names. Whistleblowing isn't a heroic blast of a trumpet; it is the lonely act of refusing to lie for a hierarchy that wouldn't hesitate to sacrifice you to save the reputation of the Trust. You are told to be a "Safety Leader," but the moment you identify a systemic defect, such as chronic understaffing, broken equipment, or the dangerous arrogance of a misguided manager, you are no longer a "team player." You are a Clinical Contaminant.

In nursing, there is no sliding scale for safety. You either hit the mark, or you fail the mission. This weight of the absolute, the full-mark requirement, is a simulator for the real world. It teaches you that in clinical practice, "almost safe" is simply unsafe. When you step into that station, you are not a student performing a script: you are a clinician managing a patient. You must find an internal rhythm of accuracy that overrides the chaos of the room.

The breakthrough occurs when you stop asking for permission to be a nurse and start acting with professional authority. When you inhabit the role with confidence, your seniors stop seeing a student and start seeing a colleague. Resilience is not a soft skill: it is written into the nursing code. Every nerve-wracking moment in that lecture theatre is an investment in your future autonomy. You are proving that you can hold your nerve while the clock is ticking and the eyes are watching.

To survive the arena, you must treat the preparation like a rehearsal for a high-stakes performance. You learn to speak your actions out loud, to narrate your safety checks, and to make your competence visible. Manifesting "I am" means accepting that you belong in that space. You have earned the right to be tested because you have survived the journey that led to the door. By the time you walk out, you are no longer the person who walked in. You have proven to the system, and more importantly to yourself, that you can be trusted with the lives of others.

The true curriculum was never just about anatomy or pharmacology: it was about the slow, deliberate construction of a professional identity.

Registration is the moment the training wheels are removed. It marks the transition from the protected student bubble to the unbuffered reality of the world of nursing. It is the moment you realise that while you were busy learning how to be a nurse, you were becoming one. As a student, you often move through the world raw, feeling every impact of the ward without the professional buffers that come with years of experience. You absorb the trauma, the noise, and the exhaustion without the shield of seniority.

The final milestone is the acquisition of your registration number. This eight-digit identifier is the ultimate symbol of your transition. You are no longer a guest in the clinical space or an observer in the chain of command. You are a standalone pillar of the national health machine. Registration is not the finish line: it is the starting block. It carries a weight of accountability that no lecture can truly describe. You have earned the right to lead because you survived the journey, the financial strain, the institutional betrayals, and the relentless sensory siege.

When that notification finally hits your inbox, the feeling is less like a victory lap and more like a tactical reset. You look at the blue uniform and realise it finally matches your level of exhaustion and your depth of knowledge. You are the final check. You are the advocate. You are the one who stands between the patient and the system. If you are currently staring at a mountain of debt and a stack of unwritten assignments, or if you are about to step into the fire for the first time, listen closely. This path will strip you back to your hardware, but rebuilding yourself into a nurse is the most high-stakes and rewarding thing you will ever do. It is not about being a hero: it is about becoming a professional who can stand in the wreckage and find a way through. You have got the grit for this.

So that was it. I was official. I had a PIN, a sense of impending doom, and a uniform that finally felt like it belonged to me. The anger and injustice I felt during training had not deterred me: it had simply refined my focus. I had the clinical skills and the professional armoury required to stay standing.

Did I survive the transition from student to newly qualified nurse, or was my core integrity double bagged and left in the sluice room for clinical collection?

For that, you will have to wait for Rookie Nurses: Buckle Up, Newly Qualified Edition to land!

Afterword

So, here we are. The stabilisers are off.

If you have made it to this page, you've survived the clinical chaos of the first three years. You've bypassed the institutional silence, lived on a budget that shouldn't legally be possible, and realised that the "hero" narrative is a cheap coat of paint used to cover up a crumbling system. You've traded your idealism for a high-grade survival instinct, and hopefully, you've kept your soul intact in the process.

But I have a secret to tell you: the stabilisers coming off isn't the end of the fear. It's just the moment the speed increases.

When I sat down to write these journals, I didn't do it to provide a "how-to" guide for passing an OSCE or writing a care plan. You have textbooks for that. I wrote this because when I was standing in those hospital corridors at 4:00 AM, I felt the crushing weight of everything we were told not to talk about. I saw the gap between the "Corporate Handshake" promised by the leadership modules and the raw, unvarnished reality of the clinical waste bin.

That gap is where Unvarnished Press (|UP| Ltd) was born.

We are a platform built for those who do the work, not those who manage it from a distance. We exist to tell the stories that usually get buried under HR policies and "professionalism" workshops. Truthful storytelling is a form of safety; it's a way to prove to the next person coming down the corridor that they aren't the only ones feeling the fire. At |UP|, we speak without the fear of reprisal, because the truth doesn't need a permit.

This book: the Student Edition, is only the first strike.

The journey from student to professional is a trilogy of survival. Very soon, the next phase of the rig will be ready for transport. In the Newly Qualified Edition, we'll look at what happens when the name on the ID badge finally carries the weight of the law, and the "protection" of the student status vanishes overnight. And finally, in the Registered Nurse Edition, we will look at the long-game: how to remain a human being in a system that views you as a shift-filler, and how to navigate the cold machinery of disciplinaries and Fitness to Practise without losing your sanity or your career.

For now, take a breath. Look at how far you've come since that first day when you couldn't even find the sluice room. You aren't a rookie anymore. You're a witness.

The ward is still there, the bleeps are still screaming, and the sharks are still circling. But now, you know how to swim.

Stay tethered to the truth. Stay unvarnished.

I'll see you in the next edition.

Victoria

Do you have a truth to tell?

|

|UP| Unvarnished Press was built on the belief that the most important stories are the ones we are told to keep quiet.

If you have a story from the healthcare front lines: the grit, the absurdity, and the reality that never makes it into the recruitment – brochures, we want to hear it. No varnish. No fear of reprisal.

Fill in the contact form on the website to join the |UP| community or submit your own "unvarnished" strike.

www.unvarnishedpress.com

|UP| The truth doesn't need a permit.

Reflective Practice Space

Reflective Practice Space

Reflective Practice Space